Multisector Casebook in Health Administration, Leadership, and Management

Multisector Casebook in Health Administration, Leadership, and Management

James A. Johnson
Central Michigan University

Scott D. Musch
Cambia Health Solutions, Inc.

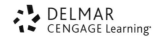

DELMAR
CENGAGE Learning·

Australia • Canada • Mexico • Singapore • Spain • United Kingdom • United States

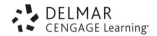

Multisector Casebook in Health Administration, Leadership, and Management
James A. Johnson and
Scott D. Musch

Vice President, Careers & Computing: Dave Garza

Director of Learning Solutions: Matt Kane

Senior Acquisitions Editor: Tari Broderick

Managing Editor: Marah Bellegarde

Associate Product Manager: Meghan E. Orvis

Editorial Assistant: Nicole Manikas

Vice President, Marketing: Jennifer Baker

Marketing Director: Wendy Mapstone

Marketing Manager: Scott Chrysler

Production Director: Wendy Troeger

Associate Product Manager: Meghan Orvis

Design and Project Management: S4Carlisle Publishing Services

Cover Design: Heidi Baughman

Cover Images:

Top: © Shutterstock/Lichtmeister

Bottom Left: © Shutterstock/kk-artworks

Bottom Middle: © Shutterstock/Feng Yu, © iStockphoto/digitalskillet

Right: © iStockphoto/Tony Tremblay

For product information and technology assistance, contact us at
Cengage Learning Customer & Sales Support, 1-800-354-9706

For permission to use material from this text or product,
submit all requests online at **www.cengage.com/permissions.**
Further permissions questions can be e-mailed to
permissionrequest@cengage.com

Example: Microsoft® is a registered trademark of the Microsoft Corporation.

Library of Congress Control Number: 2012941804

ISBN-13: 978-1-1336-0366-5

ISBN-10: 1-1336-0366-1

Delmar
5 Maxwell Drive
Clifton Park, NY 12065-2919
USA

Cengage Learning is a leading provider of customized learning solutions with office locations around the globe, including Singapore, the United Kingdom, Australia, Mexico, Brazil, and Japan. Locate your local office at: **international.cengage.com/region**

Cengage Learning products are represented in Canada by Nelson Education, Ltd.

To learn more about Delmar, visit **www.cengage.com/delmar**

Purchase any of our products at your local college store or at our preferred online store **www.cengagebrain.com**

Printed in the United States of America
1 2 3 4 5 6 7 16 15 14 13 12

Table of Contents

About the Authors

James A. Johnson, PhD, MPA, MS

Dr. Johnson teaches courses in health management and policy; organization theory and behavior; leadership; systems thinking; health administration; and community health. He has published 12 books and over 100 articles on a wide range of healthcare issues. Dr. Johnson is the past editor of the American College of Healthcare Executive's *Journal of Healthcare Management* and the Society for Human Resource Management and Organizational Behavior's *Journal of Management Practice*. He has served on many health advisory boards including the Association of University Programs in Health Administration. His work and travels have taken him to 21 different countries including work with the World Health Organization (Switzerland). He participated in field work in Africa and has lectured at Oxford University (England), University of Dublin (Ireland), University of Katmandu (Nepal), and University of Colima (Mexico). He now serves on the Scientific Advisory Board of the National Diabetes Trust Foundation (United States). Dr. Johnson was on the faculty of the Medical University of South Carolina for nearly 15 years, where he served as Chairman of the Department of Health Administration. Dr. Johnson is currently a Professor at the Dow College of Health Professions at Central Michigan University and Adjunct Professor at Auburn University and Visiting Professor at St. George's University, Grenada, West Indies.

Scott D. Musch, MBA

Mr. Musch is currently the Director of Corporate Development within the Direct Health Solutions (DHS) business of Cambia Health Solutions, Inc. Cambia's businesses include the BlueCross BlueShield health insurance plans in Oregon and Utah, and BlueShield health plans in Washington and Idaho. Mr. Musch is responsible for all aspects of the acquisition and venture investment process from deal sourcing through transaction management. Prior to joining DHS in April 2011, he was the Executive Vice President of Corporate Development for MedLink International, Inc., a healthcare information technology company. Mr. Musch has extensive experience in corporate finance, having worked in investment banking for 12 years, covering a wide variety of companies, both inside and outside the healthcare industry. Prior to joining MedLink, he was a Senior Vice President for a healthcare services focused investment bank, Shattuck Hammond Partners, a division of Morgan Keegan and Company, Inc. While at Shattuck Hammond Partners, he worked with a wide variety of healthcare payors and providers on corporate finance and business strategy matters. Prior to that, Mr. Musch worked as a Vice President in the North American

Mergers and Acquisitions Department at J.P. Morgan Securities, Inc. During his seven-year tenure at J.P. Morgan, he was actively involved in the execution and marketing of acquisitions, divestitures, strategic advisory, and private equity assignments for public and private companies in a variety of industries, including pharmaceuticals, biotech, and healthcare services. Mr. Musch earned an MBA from the Tuck School of Business at Dartmouth College, where he was a Tuck Scholar. He graduated from the University of Pennsylvania where he received a BS in Finance from the Wharton School and a BA in Economics from the College of Arts and Sciences. He is currently studying for his Doctor of Health Administration, with a graduate certificate program in International Health Services, at Central Michigan University. He is a Lean Six Sigma Green Belt in health care.

Contributors

Douglas E. Anderson, Colonel
United States Air Force
Pentagon, Virginia

James K. Arinaitwe, MPH
Candidate for MA Sustainable
Development
SIT Graduate Institute
Washington, DC

Steve Barnett, CRNA, MS
President and Chief Executive Officer
McKenzie Health System
Sandusky, Michigan

Matthew Bogner, MPH
Chief Executive Officer
Kansas Masonic Home
Wichita, Kansas

John Brady, DHA
Vice President, Physician Services
and Organizational Planning
Marianjoy Rehabilitation Hospital
Wheaton, Illinois

Judy S. Cash, MSN, MHA, RN, NE-BC
Director, GI & Perioperative Services
Baylor University Medical Center
Dallas, Texas

Frank J. Corigliano, PhD
Psychology Intern
Friends Hospital
New York, New York

Krystina Cunningham, PT, DPT
Physical Therapist
Detroit Medical Center–Rehabilitation
Institute of Michigan
Detroit, Michigan

Cheryl Daniels, RN, BSN, MSA
Assistant Director of Nursing
Dr. Susan Smith McKinney Nursing &
Rehabilitation Center
Brooklyn, New York

Anthony Drautz, RS, MSA
Environmental Health Administrator
Oakland County Health Division
Pontiac, Michigan

Tracy J. Farnsworth, MHSA, MBA
Interim Director and Associate Dean
Kasiska School of Health Professions
Division of Health Sciences
Idaho State University
Pocatello, Idaho

Deymon X. Fleming, MPH
Principal Management Official
Centers for Disease Control
and Prevention
Atlanta, Georgia

Andrea Frederick, RN, MSN
Assistant Professor of Nursing
Saginaw Valley State University
University Center, Michigan

Jessica Gardon Rose, PA, MEd
Director, Carls Center for Clinical Care &
Education
Clinical Instructor
Central Michigan University
College of Health Professions
Mount Pleasant, Michigan

Cynthia E. Harris, DHA, MBPA, MSW
Assistant Professor & Special Assistant
for Academic and Student Advancement
Howard University School of Social Work
Washington, DC

Patrick M. Hermanson, DHA
Program Director, Health Care
Administration
Idaho State University
Pocatello, Idaho

James Allen Johnson III, MPH
Research Assistant
Jiann-Ping Hsu College of Public Health
Georgia Southern University
Statesboro, Georgia

**Sharon Williams Lewis, DHA,
RN-BC, CPM**
Program Manager
District of Columbia Department
of Health
Health Regulations and Licensing
Administration
Health Care Facilities Division
Washington, DC

Genesa L. Mays, MSA
Director of Perioperative Services
Owens & Minor
Mechanicsville, Virginia

David Meckstroth, MBA
Consultant
Meck Consulting, LLC
Troy, Ohio

James Christopher Middlebrook, DHA
Chief Executive Officer
Helping Hands Home Assistance, Inc.
Knoxville, Tennessee

Adam Miller, MPA
Director, State Health Policy
Astellas US LLC
Canton, Michigan

Asal Mohamadi, PhD
Visiting Professor
Center for International Affairs
Georgia Southern University
Statesboro, Georgia

Domingo J. Navarro, MBA
STD/HIV and TB Program
San Antonio Metropolitan Health District
San Antonio, Texas

**Margaret Ozan Rafferty, MBA,
MHA, RN**
Managing Director
OzanPartners, LLC
Orland Park, Illinois

Stanley A. Phillip, Jr., MHA
Deputy Branch Chief
Centers for Disease Control
and Prevention
Prevention Program Branch,
NCHHSTP/DHAP
Atlanta, Georgia

David J. Ranney, MBA, MIM
Private Consultant
Post Falls, Idaho

Kathleen M. Reville, MEd
Senior Vice President/Chief
Program Officer
Seven Hills Foundation
Worcester, Massachusetts

James E. Selby, Jr., MPA
Supervisory Management Officer
Office of Translational Sciences, Center
for Drug Evaluation and Research
Food and Drug Administration
Silver Spring, Maryland

Ben Spedding, MA, NCC
Part-Time Faculty, Psychology Program
School of Undergraduate Studies
Capella University
Minneapolis, Minnesota

Beth Ann Taylor, RN, MBA, NEA-BC
Associate Director for Patient Care Services
Clement J. Zablocki VA Medical Center
Milwaukee, Wisconsin

Catherine Vyskocil-Maxwell, RN, BSN, MA
Executive Director, Advocacy Officer
St. Joseph Health System
Tawas City, Michigan

Kay Wagner, MSN, RN
Director of Quality
MidMichigan Health
Midland, Michigan

Emily van de Water, PT, DPT
Physical Therapist
San Mateo Medical Center
San Mateo, California

Victor D. Weeden, CDFM
Medical Clinic Administrator
RAF Croughton, England

Andrew Westrum, DHA, MBA
Program Manager, Nurse Advice Line
TRICARE Management Activity
Office of the Chief Medical Officer
Falls Church, Virginia

Kevin Wiley, Jr., MPH
Health Policy and Management Student
Jiann-Ping Hsu College of Public Health
Georgia Southern University
Statesboro, Georgia

William G. Wuenstel, MBA, RN, CCRN
Director Critical Care Department
Munroe Regional Health System
Ocala, Florida

INTRODUCTION

The case-study method brings interesting, real-world experiences into the classroom. Case scenarios expose students to management roles and responsibilities. They provide students with the opportunity to assume varying roles within case situations and reflect on the different perspectives of the characters involved. One benefit of the case-study method is students learn to understand in professional and managerial situations that there are no clear-cut right and wrong decisions. Students often need and want guidance to find the "right decision." In management, however, many times no right decision exists, but rather decisions that may be better than others given a particular set of circumstances. Often, decisions are dictated by policies or code, such as legal, ethical, or organizational regulations. Decisions that have a clear outcome on the basis of these policies are often rare in practice. More often, professionals must balance competing stakeholder interests that offer no clear-cut resolutions. Within these types of predicaments lie the real challenge for managers and leaders. Experience, reflection, and consultation of others are the necessary guides for reaching effective outcomes. As students work through these case scenarios, they will gain an understanding of such competencies for making quality decisions. They will develop the ability to think through how to approach challenging situations, analyze the issues and assumptions involved, consider stakeholder concerns, and make comprehensive and fair recommendations.

The case scenarios presented in this book provide a foundation for analyzing critical issues facing healthcare leaders today. They reflect the myriad of situations that occur within the various subsectors of the healthcare industry, including hospitals, health insurance plans, medical groups, public health organizations, governmental agencies, pharmaceutical companies, and many others. In writing cases, an author is faced with the challenge of narrowing down the universe of possible management scenarios into a collection that is at both times comprehensive and manageable. The cases in this book aim to capture "real-life" scenarios in real or fictional healthcare settings. They were written to reinforce the understanding of and to stimulate creative thinking about the many nuances of management in the healthcare sector. Their scope involves professionals at varying levels of authority in a wide range of roles and organizations, both inside and outside the healthcare industry. The names of the characters, organizations, and settings have been fictionalized, unless otherwise noted. The case scenarios are intended for teaching and discussion purposes only.

Case-Study Approach

Students will find many sources available on how to analyze a case scenario and the elements to include in a written or oral report. The purpose here is to highlight a few features to enhance the case-study approach.

Case scenarios often leave out complete information. This is a deliberate strategy by the author. Managers and leaders often have to make decisions in a context of incomplete information. This is decision making in a real-world environment. Students should learn to seek out additional information efficiently and effectively. This involves learning both what pertinent questions to ask to collect the right information and how to gather such information. Time constraints in the decision-making process require managers to learn to define a problem precisely and recognize the essential information necessary to reach a solution. Students should understand the importance of making reasonable assumptions in the case scenario and being flexible to modify those assumptions to different iterations of character and event interactions. Moreover, students should recognize that in the case-study method, their analytical method in reaching a decision is often just as important as the actual solution. No prescribed solutions are offered in these cases. This enables instructors to have the flexibility to focus on particular lessons or objectives within each case.

At the end of each case scenario are discussion questions specific to that case to consider. In addition, the student may benefit by reflecting on the broader issues inherent within the case and how such issues may affect decision making. Some larger considerations might include:

- What factors—history, culture, politics, environment, organizational structure, communication, and character attributes—contributed to the problem or success of the situation?

- Identify all the stakeholders affected by the current scenario. Identify additional stakeholders who may become involved after implementation of the decision.

- What are all of the issues involved in the case? Do the issues require different and potentially contradictory decisions?

- How does the context of the scenario facilitate or inhibit decision making?

- How does the type of organization involved in the case influence or drive the particular circumstances of the situation described?

- What are the likely short-term and long-term consequences of the decision?

- Evaluate the temperature level of the decision response. Is it appropriate for the current situation or might it raise the temperature (e.g., is the professional underreacting or overreacting)?

- Does the professional have support of key stakeholders for the decision or will the situation involve building allies?

- What is the appropriate timing of the decision response? When is the best time to pull the trigger? Does the situation require immediate action or is there time for reflection and consultation?

- What is the professional's level of authority? Does the decision require prior approval of senior management or does the professional have the necessary authority to execute the decision on his or her own?

- How will the decision affect the organization's external environment?

As students work through these case scenarios, they should try to resolve the immediate management situation, but also should aim to serve a greater role and responsibility. Healthcare professionals should strive for leadership. In doing so, students should reflect on the different roles implicit in any given situation as they develop recommendations for the cases.

- Professional: Works within the boundaries of his/her job description and responsibilities, successfully executes his/her duties.

- Manager: Supervises professionals in carrying out their job responsibilities to ensure successful and timely completion to accomplish an organization's goals; focuses on efficient and effective execution; works within boundaries established by role.

- Leader: Assumes role beyond immediate management goals and questions effectiveness of existing roles and responsibilities to achieve a strategic goal or objective; thinks "outside the box" to develop solutions; moves beyond existing boundaries to ensure goals and strategy are aligned properly to succeed in a dynamic environment.

The case scenarios in this book will assist students to think through important management concepts and help augment their skills to fulfill effectively their responsibilities as healthcare professionals, managers, and as students striving for leadership roles in the industry.

Structure

The case scenarios in this book are related to the major branches of management: strategic management, financial management, human resource management (encompasses organizational behavior management), program planning and implementation (substitutes for marketing management), operations management, information systems (technology) management, quality improvement and service management, and communication management. In addition to these traditional management topics, we included professional ethics. Table 1–1 categorizes the cases according to the main management topics covered in the cases. Table 1–2 categorizes the cases according to the healthcare organizations involved in the scenarios. These matrices should help guide instructors and students in integrating the cases into their coursework.

Table 1–1 Relationship between Cases and Management Topics

	Strategic Planning and Management	Financial Management	Human Resource Management	Program Planning and Implementation	Operations Management	Information Systems Management	Quality Improvement and Service Management	Communication Management	Professional Ethics
Case 1: Selling a Medicaid Managed Care Company	•								
Case 2: Independent Medical Practices—Becoming Extinct?	•								
Case 3: Strategic Options Assessment for a Catholic Health System's Health Plan	•								
Case 4: The Mission Discernment Process	•								
Case 5: Rural Healthcare Development under Healthcare Reform	•				○			○	
Case 6: A Change in Culture at a CCRC	•				○		○		
Case 7: Addressing the Psychological Effects of Exposure to Community Violence	•			•					
Case 8: Leadership—New Team, New Initiative	•		○		○				
Case 9: Dropping Small-Group Insurance Products		•		○					
Case 10: Managing Retail-Based Health Clinics: Financial Performance and Mission	○	•			○				
Case 11: Rural Medical Practice—Balancing Needs and Necessities		•		○					
Case 12: How Do You End an Unprofitable Business Relationship?	○	•							
Case 13: Budget Cuts in a Home Care Program		•						○	
Case 14: When One Collaborative Member Threatens to End Financial Support		•			•				
Case 15: FQHC—A Cure for Ailing Community Health Centers?	○	•							
Case 16: Nonprofit Losing Funding, Not Faith		•							
Case 17: Beyond a Patient Complaint		•						○	
Case 18: Building Latrines—Half the Solution to Global Sanitation		•		•	○			○	

Legend: • = directly related   ○ = indirectly related

Continues

Table 1–1 (Continued)

	Strategic Planning and Management	Financial Management	Human Resource Management	Program Planning and Implementation	Operations Management	Information Systems Management	Quality Improvement and Service Management	Communication Management	Professional Ethics
Case 19: Numbers and Degrees—Challenges for the Nursing Workforce	•		•						
Case 20: Orienting a Contract Physical Therapist			•						
Case 21: Revamping Ineffective Performance Reviews			•						
Case 22: We, the Counselors			•					○	
Case 23: A Case of Reverse Discrimination?			•						
Case 24: Sexual Harassment at St. Catherine			•						
Case 25: Understanding Millennial Employees			•					○	
Case 26: Managing Diversity			•					○	
Case 27: Broken Promises			•						
Case 28: Sick Building Syndrome			•		○				○
Case 29: Don't Ask, But Tell			•		○				○
Case 30: Top Ten U.S. Public Health Achievements			•	○					
Case 31: Tuberculosis in the Workplace			•						○
Case 32: Zero Tolerance for Smoking			•	•					
Case 33: Ethiopia's Struggle with Resource Management			•	•	○			○	
Case 34: The Family Health Initiative				•	○				
Case 35: The Anti-Vaccination Paradigm				•				○	
Case 36: Collaborative Approach to Diabetes Prevention and Care	○	○		•					
Case 37: Healthy Lifestyles Start at Home				•				○	
Case 38: Transition Planning for Foster Youth with Special Health Care Needs	○			•			○		

Legend: • = directly related   ○ = indirectly related

Continues

Table 1–1 (Continued)

	Strategic Planning and Management	Financial Management	Human Resource Management	Program Planning and Implementation	Operations Management	Information Systems Management	Quality Improvement and Service Management	Communication Management	Professional Ethics
Case 39: Community Coalitions and the Built Environment				•				○	
Case 40: Medical Care Taking Flight	○			•			○		
Case 41: Rural Health Care in Central Michigan	○	○	○	•				○	
Case 42: Smoking Cessation Program Implementation				•	○				
Case 43: The Unexpected Problems			○		•				
Case 44: Simplifying an Organizational Chart			○		•				
Case 45: Launching into the "New Normal"	○			○	•			○	
Case 46: Journey to Discharge				○	•		○		
Case 47: Team Collaboration in Delivering Integrated Systems of Care					•		○	○	
Case 48: Syphilis Outbreak Response in Puerto Rico					•			○	
Case 49: Pacific Needle Exchange Program				○	•				
Case 50: Post-EHR Implementation—The Recovery Room Slowdown						•	•		
Case 51: Go or No Go—An Executive's Information System Dilemma	○	○				•			
Case 52: Electronic Environmental Health Program Management Tool					○	•			
Case 53: Building a Better Budget Tracking System		○				•			
Case 54: Adverse Events in a Postanesthesia Care Unit			○		○			•	
Case 55: Unacceptable Backlogs in the Sterile Processing Department			○		○			•	
Case 56: Responsibility in the Development of a Pressure Ulcer								•	○

Legend: • = directly related   ○ = indirectly related

Continues

Table 1–1 (Continued)

	Strategic Planning and Management	Financial Management	Human Resource Management	Program Planning and Implementation	Operations Management	Information Systems Management	Quality Improvement and Service Management	Communication Management	Professional Ethics
Case 57: Recurring Mistake			•				•		
Case 58: HIV Testing at a Health and Fitness Fair							•	○	
Case 59: To Hear This Message in Korean, Press 9					○		•	•	
Case 60: Blackout 2003—An Environmental Health Response					○		•	•	
Case 61: Communicating the Need for Hospital Consolidation	○	○			○			•	
Case 62: A *Giardia* Outbreak?								•	○
Case 63: Senior Cyber Café			•				○	•	
Case 64: Toy Recall Prompts Attention to Lead Poisoning							○	•	
Case 65: A Communications Challenge								•	
Case 66: Ethical Limits of Patient Satisfaction			○				○	○	•
Case 67: Neglected Tropical Diseases—A Local NGO's Challenges		○			○				•
Case 68: A Friend's Dilemma			○						•
Case 69: Stolen Briefcase							○		•
Case 70: Theatre of Operation—Transplant Solutions in Public Health				○				○	•
Case 71: Role of Public Health in End-of-Life Issues				○				○	•

Legend: • = directly related   ○ = indirectly related

Table 1–2 Relationship between Cases and Healthcare Organizations

	Private Nonprofit	Private / Public For-Profit	Government			
			Federal	State	Local	International
Case 1: Selling a Medicaid Managed Care Company	•					
Case 2: Independent Medical Practices—Becoming Extinct?		•				
Case 3: Strategic Options Assessment for a Catholic Health System's Health Plan	•					
Case 4: The Mission Discernment Process	•					
Case 5: Rural Healthcare Development under Healthcare Reform	•					
Case 6: A Change in Culture at a CCRC		•				
Case 7: Addressing the Psychological Effects of Exposure to Community Violence	•					
Case 8: Leadership—New Team, New Initiative			•			
Case 9: Dropping Small-Group Insurance Products		•				
Case 10: Managing Retail-Based Health Clinics: Financial Performance and Mission		•				
Case 11: Rural Medical Practice—Balancing Needs and Necessities		•				
Case 12: How Do You End an Unprofitable Business Relationship?		•				
Case 13: Budget Cuts in a Home Care Program				○	•	
Case 14: When One Collaborative Member Threatens to End Financial Support	•					
Case 15: FQHC—A Cure for Ailing Community Health Centers?	•		○			
Case 16: Nonprofit Losing Funding, Not Faith	•					
Case 17: Beyond a Patient Complaint	•		○			
Case 18: Building Latrines—Half the Solution to Global Sanitation	•					
Case 19: Numbers and Degrees—Challenges for the Nursing Workforce	•					
Case 20: Orienting a Contract Physical Therapist		•				

Legend: • = directly related   ○ = indirectly related

© Cengage Learning 2013

Continues

Table 1–2 *(Continued)*

	Private Nonprofit	Private / Public For-Profit	Government			
			Federal	State	Local	International
Case 21: Revamping Ineffective Performance Reviews	•					
Case 22: We, the Counselors	•					
Case 23: A Case of Reverse Discrimination?	•					
Case 24: Sexual Harassment at St. Catherine	•					
Case 25: Understanding Millennial Employees				•		
Case 26: Managing Diversity					•	
Case 27: Broken Promises	•					
Case 28: Sick Building Syndrome		•	○			
Case 29: Don't Ask, But Tell			•			
Case 30: Top Ten U.S. Public Health Achievements			•			
Case 31: Tuberculosis in the Workplace					•	
Case 32: Zero Tolerance for Smoking	•			○		
Case 33: Ethiopia's Struggle with Resource Management	○					•
Case 34: The Family Health Initiative			•			
Case 35: The Anti-Vaccination Paradigm					•	
Case 36: Collaborative Approach to Diabetes Prevention and Care	•	•	○			
Case 37: Healthy Lifestyles Start at Home	•					
Case 38: Transition Planning for Foster Youth with Special Health Care Needs				○	•	
Case 39: Community Coalitions and the Built Environment				•	•	
Case 40: Medical Care Taking Flight		•				
Case 41: Rural Health Care in Central Michigan	•			•	•	
Case 42: Smoking Cessation Program Implementation	•					
Case 43: The Unexpected Problems		•				

Legend: • = directly related   ○ = indirectly related

Continues

Table 1–2 *(Continued)*

	Private Nonprofit	Private / Public For-Profit	Government			
			Federal	State	Local	International
Case 44: Simplifying an Organizational Chart		•				
Case 45: Launching into the "New Normal"		•				
Case 46: Journey to Discharge	•					
Case 47: Team Collaboration in Delivering Integrated Systems of Care	•					
Case 48: Syphilis Outbreak Response in Puerto Rico			o			•
Case 49: Pacific Needle Exchange Program	•			o		
Case 50: Post-EHR Implementation—The Recovery Room Slowdown		•				
Case 51: Go or No Go—An Executive's Information System Dilemma		•				
Case 52: Electronic Environmental Health Program Management Tool				•	•	
Case 53: Building a Better Budget Tracking System			•			
Case 54: Adverse Events in a Postanesthesia Care Unit		•				
Case 55: Unacceptable Backlogs in the Sterile Processing Department	•					
Case 56: Responsibility in the Development of a Pressure Ulcer		•				
Case 57: Recurring Mistake	•					
Case 58: HIV Testing at a Health and Fitness Fair					•	
Case 59: To Hear This Message in Korean, Press 9	•					
Case 60: Blackout 2003—An Environmental Health Response				o	•	
Case 61: Communicating the Need for Hospital Consolidation	•					
Case 62: A *Giardia* Outbreak?				•	o	
Case 63: Senior Cyber Café	•					
Case 64: Toy Recall Prompts Attention to Lead Poisoning		o	•	•		
Case 65: A Communications Challenge	•					

Legend: • = directly related   o = indirectly related

Continues

Table 1–2 *(Continued)*

	Private Nonprofit	Private / Public For-Profit	Government			
			Federal	State	Local	International
Case 66: Ethical Limits of Patient Satisfaction		•				
Case 67: Neglected Tropical Diseases—A Local NGO's Challenges	•					•
Case 68: A Friend's Dilemma				•	•	
Case 69: Stolen Briefcase				•		
Case 70: Theatre of Operation—Transplant Solutions in Public Health		o		•		
Case 71: Role of Public Health in End-of-Life Issues	•					

Legend: • = directly related   o = indirectly related

Summary of Common Themes

Across the case scenarios, regardless of responsibility level or organization type, common themes appear that are instructive "takeaways" for professionals in health care.

1. *Engage stakeholders in the decision-making process.* At the beginning of a problem or opportunity, the healthcare professional should identify all stakeholders affected and take the time to understand their primary concerns. Managers need to involve key stakeholders during the process. Managers can learn from the diverse perspectives of stakeholders and at the same time ensure that their concerns are being addressed. By including stakeholders at the appropriate time and level in the decision-making process, a manager can gain their support in implementing and accepting a tough decision.

2. *Learn to effectively work in and manage teams.* Teamwork is a critical component within health care. The workforce in the healthcare industry is highly educated and eager to participate in the decision-making process that affects them and the long-term interests of the organizations they serve. The benefits of a team approach are too numerous to list, but they primarily involve integrating the diversity of experiences, skills, and perspectives of team members to reach an optimal work product. The development and operation of productive teams require a skill set gained through education and experience. Important considerations include team member selection, size, diversity, type, and structure.

3. *Be in front of a problem or opportunity.* Managers need to ensure that the appropriate organizational structures are in place to assist professionals and staff to make sound decisions in the first place. It takes less time, energy, and costs to prevent a problem from emerging than it does to fix a problem once it occurs. Likewise, having structures in place will enable an organization to seize on an opportunity, exemplifying the old adage "Prepare for an opportunity, rather than wait for an opportunity to prepare."

4. *Learn to communicate effectively.* Aside from having proficient communication skills, managers need to recognize when to communicate. There are several stages at which to apply effective communication in a decision-making process. At the beginning of any process, the manager should make sure everyone has a clear understanding of roles, responsibilities, and expectations, and that they are openly receptive to questions and concerns. During the process, the manager should offer guidance and seek feedback along the way to avoid any surprises at the end. Lastly, at the end, the manager should take the time to seek constructive feedback and share lessons learned. Every scenario presents an excellent learning opportunity.

5. *Embrace systems thinking.* Systems thinking has become a necessary competency for healthcare professionals. We live and operate within systems. Interconnections, relationships, and interdependencies affect health behaviors and the performance of policies and programs aimed at addressing key concerns. Leaders in the healthcare industry need to embrace systems thinking and learn to realize the many complexities inherent in a systems-wide approach.

6. *Recognize and embrace diverse backgrounds.* The scope of the healthcare industry is vast, encompassing a wide range of specialist and generalist areas, clinical and nonclinical expertise, and drawing on a large diversity of professional backgrounds and talents. Managers need to value this diversity. They should incorporate the wealth of experiences and perspectives within their programs and organizations.

7. *Remember health care is largely a service industry.* At the core of all service industries are people. In all professions dedicated to serving people, managers will encounter human fallacies. It is to be expected, but it should not deter managers as it can also be a great source of inspiration and creativity. Healthcare professionals need to recognize that human behavior cannot be modeled or anticipated. They cannot plan for every contingency. They need to be prepared to encounter and embrace this human dimension of health care.

8. *Embrace your role as a professional.* It should be the role of each individual employee to take responsibility to uphold an organization's mission and standards. It does not serve anyone in the long run to defer this responsibility to someone else, to another manager or otherwise. Professionalism requires resisting the temptation to just "get the job done" or to fall back on the old "it's not my responsibility" response. Professionals should not let opportunities slip away. Take the time to communicate, motivate, evaluate, coordinate, educate, and most important, lead.

9. *Sustain the mission of health care.* The case scenarios presented in this book illustrate the far-reaching aspects of the healthcare industry and the primary mission to promote the health and safety of all citizens. Health care touches so many dimensions of our daily lives. In fulfilling their job responsibilities, healthcare professionals serve not only the immediate purposes of their organizations, but the greater overall mission of health care. They embrace the opportunities to have a significant effect on people's lives and make a difference in the future health and well-being of our global community.

PART

II

CASES

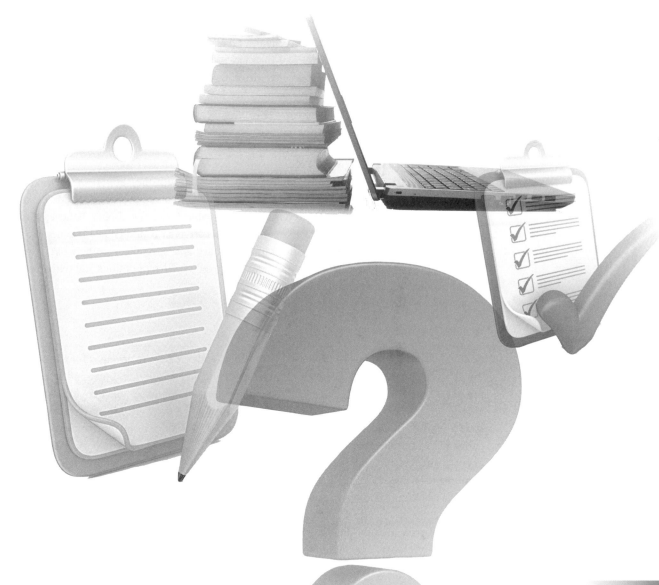

Case 1

Selling a Medicaid Managed Care Company

CASE CONTRIBUTOR Scott D. Musch

Situation

Sunlight Health Plan ("Sunlight" or the "Plan") is an independent, not-for-profit managed care company dedicated to serving the needs of low- and moderate-income residents in Kings County, New York. Sunlight is a prepaid health services plan ("PHSP") with a membership base consisting of residents enrolled in Medicaid Managed Care ("Medicaid"), Child Health Plus ("CHP"), or Family Health Plus ("FHP"). The Plan is one of only several PHSPs operating in its county. The Plan has the highest Medicaid membership in the county and has experienced gains and declines consistent with the overall Medicaid membership market. Given its mandate, the Plan has had to limit its enrollment to Medicaid eligibles in its direct service area. The Plan's lack of scale creates relatively high administrative costs that cannot be spread out over an expanding membership base. In addition, New York's complex regulatory environment further affects the Plan's ability to secure contracts with specialty providers.

Consequently, the president of Sunlight, Dr. Lopez, with the support of the Plan's board of trustees, has decided to pursue a sale of the Plan to a larger operator of Medicaid managed care plans, subject to agreement of acceptable terms. Dr. Lopez believes that transferring the Plan's members to a larger managed care plan would enable the members to access a broader geographically diversified primary and specialty care network. This additional access should translate into overall improved healthcare options and outcomes, and lower medical and administrative costs.

Background

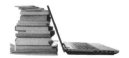

Sunlight began operations in 1990 as a Medicaid provider. The Plan arranges for the delivery of healthcare services to persons eligible for Medicaid and provides other public health programs for low-income families and individuals. Beyond Medicaid, the Plan offers CHP, a program for low-income, uninsured children, and FHP, a program for low-income, uninsured adults. Medicaid, CHP, and FHP are referred to as "Government Sponsored Programs." As of December 31, 2011, the Plan had 11,000 Medicaid members (including unborns), 4000 CHP members, and 300 FHP members. Sunlight has the largest Medicaid enrollment in its service area. The Plan contracts with federally qualified health centers (FQHCs) including county-owned primary care centers and hospital-sponsored health centers (collectively "Health Centers"). These Health Centers serve as the sole providers of primary care services for the Plan. In addition, the Plan offers specialty care through more than 1000 specialists. Given Sunlight's relative size, the Plan contracts with a company to provide billing and claims processing, administrative services, and management information systems, including reports on membership, providers, specialists, hospitals, financial management, and other member services.

The Plan, as well as all New York State Medicaid plans, has been under a rate freeze from the Department of Health for Medicaid and FHP. A minor escalator for emergency room services and maternity-related services was recently granted. It is expected that in the next year or two, Medicaid plans will receive a trend increase combined with a risk-adjusted rate increase. The Plan's consolidated medical loss ratio has averaged 87% during the last four years. The Plan's administrative loss ratio has ranged from a low of 13% to a high of 18% during that same period, making the Plan breakeven at best.

Sunlight's primary focus has been on its constituents, which include its members, providers, and state regulators. The Plan consistently strives to provide excellent service to its three primary constituent groups, Medicaid, CHP, and FHP members. The Plan's participating Health Centers and providers have strong ties to the communities they serve, and along with the Plan's marketing and community outreach show a proven commitment to provide high quality, culturally sensitive, and logistically accessible health care. This affiliation with the Health Centers is perceived as a benefit, since it offers patients a single site for routine diagnosis, testing, and treatment. The Plan provides a comprehensive range of healthcare benefits as required by the Medicaid, CHP, and FHP programs. While the specific scope of benefits varies by program, the basic benefits include primary and preventive care, specialty services, inpatient hospitalization, urgent and emergency care, and behavioral health and substance abuse treatment services. Certain services, including pharmacy, dental, and behavioral health utilization review services, are provided through subcontracting relationships with third parties.

Managed care has become the dominant delivery system for New York's government sponsored programs. Two of these programs, FHP and CHP, are exclusively managed care programs with no fee-for-service option. While the New York State Medicaid program retains a fee-for-service option for certain consumers under some limited conditions, enrollment in managed care is mandatory for the vast majority of Medicaid beneficiaries in the state. Medicaid is the basic New York State program for those who cannot afford to pay for medical care. Eligibility is determined based on net monthly income and available financial resources, and varies with the number of individuals in the family unit. It includes all primary care, most specialist services, hospital, emergency room, vision, dental, outpatient, behavioral health, and pharmacy. A Medicaid-eligible individual or family must meet the mandated income, resource, age, and/or disability requirements to qualify.

Next Steps

In preparing the Plan for a potential sale, Dr. Lopez prepared a market analysis of the most likely parties who would be interested in exploring an acquisition of Sunlight. The obvious choices would be competing health plans. There are five other competitors in the county market that provide Medicaid, CHP, and FHP programs. All of these competitors have significantly larger membership statewide than Sunlight, but the Plan has the largest Medicaid membership in the county. Competitors include provider-sponsored (i.e., hospital), private, and publicly-traded companies. In addition, other private and publicly-traded companies who are seeking market entry into the county or New York State might be interested. There are many companies that fall into this category.

In discussions with his legal counsel, Dr. Lopez understands that a proposed transaction will be structured as a sale or assignment of assets and the assumption of associated provider contracts, or a membership substitution if the acquirer is also a nonprofit. To ensure continuity of primary care services, Dr. Lopez anticipates that the acquirer of the Plan will enter into (or assume the Plan's existing) provider agreements with the Health Centers for a mutually acceptable period of time, if the acquirer does not already have provider agreements with these Health Centers in place. In addition, as part of a proposed transaction, Dr. Lopez wants an all-cash offer and an administrative arrangement for the payment of Incurred But Not Reported ("IBNR") claims after closing. Even with all of these considerations, Dr. Lopez recognizes that any transaction ultimately will be subject to the approval of the New York regulatory authorities.

Discussion Questions

1. What factors do you think led to Dr. Lopez and the board of trustees' decision to sell Sunlight Health Plan?

2. What characteristics make the Plan an attractive acquisition opportunity for an experienced Medicaid managed care organization?

3. What factors should Dr. Lopez and the board consider in selecting a potential acquirer?

4. Why would Dr. Lopez want the acquirer to either enter into new, or assume the existing, provider agreements with the Health Centers? What considerations does this require of a purchaser? How might it affect transaction timing?

5. Why does Dr. Lopez want an administrative arrangement for the payment of IBNR claims after closing? How does IBNR affect the purchase price of a transaction?

6. What factors might influence the decision of New York regulatory authorities to approve one potential acquirer of the Plan over another?

Case 2

Independent Medical Practices— Becoming Extinct?

CASE CONTRIBUTOR **Scott D. Musch**

Situation

Dr. Sue Jensen and Dr. Emily Gilsan own Woodland Family Practice (Woodland), an independent primary care practice located outside of Tacoma, Washington. Dr. Jensen moved to Tacoma 10 years ago and started Woodland as a solo family practice in the community. Although she had options to join larger medical groups and clinics after medical school, she chose to establish her own medical practice in order to have autonomy and build stronger patient relationships in the community. The patient-payor mix for the practice has been consistently divided among commercial insurance and Medicare. She is a participating provider in Medicare. In addition, she sees Medicaid patients occasionally and helps those who are uninsured on a pro bono basis. As her practice developed, Dr. Jensen needed to bring in another physician to help support the practice and patient load. She contacted a former classmate, Dr. Gilsan, and encouraged her to join Woodland several years ago as a co-owner.

As a two-physician practice, however, Woodland has not been able to generate enough cash to invest meaningfully back into the business. For instance, the practice needs to hire a nurse case manager, implement an electronic health record (EHR) system that qualifies for meaningful use, and add a patient portal to its website. Woodland would need to take out a sizable bank loan if the physicians wanted to make such investments. Dr. Jensen and Dr. Gilsan are concerned that as healthcare reform unfolds and the market continues to evolve, operating as a two-physician, independent practice will become increasingly difficult. As accountable care organizations and patient-centered medical homes (PCMHs) advance in the market, small independent practices will be at a relative disadvantage without enhanced capabilities.

Background

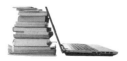

The number of small physician practices has been declining over the last decade, with a growing number of physicians working in large group practices, hospitals, or other medical settings (see Table 2–1). Although this decline reflects broader economic trends, it also indicates the financial realities of practicing medicine on a smaller scale. Reimbursement rates for Medicare and third-party payors continue to be slashed or, at best, temporarily frozen. Small practices have little negotiating power in negotiating insurance contracts compared to larger groups, and often have to take whatever reimbursement rates they are offered in their contracts.

Table 2–1 Physicians in Solo/Two-Physician Practices vs. All Other Practice Settings

	Solo/Two-Physician Practices	All Other Practice Settings
1996–97	40.7%	59.3%
1998–99	37.5%	62.6%
2000–01	35.2%	64.8%
2004–05	32.5%	67.5%

Source: *"Physicians Moving to Mid-Sized, Single-Specialty Practices," by A. Liebhaber and J. M. Grossman, August 2007,* Center for Studying Health System Change, *p. 1.*[1]

Small practices will be at a relative disadvantage in the market for accountable care arrangements. In order for accountable care organizations to succeed in providing better care at lower costs, participants need to use data more effectively to manage patient populations. Physicians also need to have the time and ability to reach out to patients and monitor their conditions, which requires a whole level of new physician-patient engagement. These capabilities require enhancements in technology and staffing; capabilities that small practices, like Woodland, cannot afford. Practices that have become accredited as PCMHs have an edge in this respect as they have been using EHRs already to collect and analyze the health of patient populations. Although Woodland has been evaluating the investment involved in becoming accredited as a PCMH, it is a long way from having the money necessary to buy the technology and hire the staff to meet the requirements. As a result, Woodland is unprepared to accept greater financial risk for managing patient care.

Next Steps

Dr. Jensen and Dr. Gilsan have been evaluating their strategic options for Woodland. They have thought long and hard about the many alternatives available to them, particularly given all the news releases over the last year of decisions of other independent practices to sell or join other groups. After considerable discussion, they have developed a list of potential strategic options for Woodland.

- Sell to a hospital/health system (integrated model). Several large hospital systems in the Seattle/Tacoma market are actively acquiring small physician practices. One of the main reasons hospitals acquire independent practices is to bring their patients into the hospital network, which can be a major source of additional revenue through referrals for hospital inpatient and outpatient services.
- Sell to/merge with a large medical group. Larger medical groups are typically multispecialty and have around 50 or more physicians. There are a limited number in Woodland's immediate service area.
- Join an independent physician association (IPA). The market has few well-organized IPAs and most lack the scale of similar types of organizations in larger markets, such as Hill Physicians Medical Group and Brown & Toland Physicians in the San Francisco Bay area. IPAs exist to help independent practices survive and flourish. They provide help with managed care insurance contracting, clinical

care coordination, technology implementation, health information exchange, data analytics, and billing and administrative services.

- Convert to a concierge or retainer model. In this type of model, the physicians would provide a greater level of service for a limited number of patients, such as offering on-demand, 24/7 access. These patients would pay a monthly or annual fee to Woodland to provide this service. Current industry examples include PartnerMD, LLC (www.partnermd.com), MDVIP, Inc. (www.mdvip.com), and One Medical Group, Inc. (www.onemedical.com).

- Recruit additional physicians to expand Woodland. Becoming a larger practice and achieving some economies of scale could enable Woodland to generate more cash, which could be invested back into the practice.

- Hire a third-party services company that could offer the practice a turnkey solution to gain PCMH capabilities. Companies such as TransforMED (www.transformed .com) and RiseHealth, Inc. (www.risehealth.com) offer a menu of services, including change management consultants, technology, and other resources, to transform primary care practices into more economically viable businesses.

- Status quo. Under this option, the physicians are making a bet that health insurance payors will start to reimburse primary care physicians more for their services. It assumes that payors will value the higher level of patient care coordination (as in PCMHs) that primary care practices could offer.

Discussion Questions

1. Evaluate the pros and cons for each strategic alternative. Consider the short-term as well as long-term implications of each option.

2. What are the professional and financial incentives of each option for the physicians?

3. One criticism of the integrated model is that physicians, as hospital employees, lose a level of engagement that can result in a drop in revenue for the hospital. How can a hospital incent employed physicians to feel more responsibility for financial performance?

4. How will the healthcare industry be affected by the decline in the number of small physician practices?

5. What strategic option would you recommend for Woodland?

Reference

[1] Liebhaber, A., & Grossman, J. M. (2007, August). *Physicians moving to mid-sized, single-specialty practices* (Tracking Report No. 18). Retrieved from Center for Studying Health System Change at http://www.hschange.com/CONTENT/941/?words=solo%20practices

Case 3

Strategic Options Assessment for a Catholic Health System's Health Plan

CASE CONTRIBUTOR **Scott D. Musch**

Situation

St. Mary's Health System (SMHS) is a nonprofit Catholic healthcare ministry committed to providing for the needs of the communities it serves, especially for those who are poor and vulnerable. SMHS began more than 100 years ago and continues its tradition of caring that was started by the Franciscan Sisters of Mary. SMHS's comprehensive scope of services includes 10 hospitals, physician clinics, home health programs, senior services, and a health plan. The health system operates in four states in the Midwest.

Since its inception in 1985, SMHS's health plan, called Healthy Lives, has focused on providing health maintenance organization (HMO) products. Healthy Lives has a long-standing reputation for superb care and quality service. The health plan has received the National Committee of Quality Assurance's (NCQA) highest rating of "Excellent" for the past five years and has also obtained the highest member satisfaction ratings of health plans in its regional market. The management team of Healthy Lives has been committed to providing the highest quality care possible and maintaining outstanding customer service ratings.

Historically, Healthy Lives has focused on providing a traditional HMO product. However, recent industry and market trends have forced management to focus on a product diversification strategy. As employers continue to seek low-cost products to reduce benefit expenses, demand for high-deductible plans has grown. As a result, Healthy Lives recently added a high-deductible HMO product as part of its diversification strategy. In addition, the health plan added consumer-driven health plan (CDHP) features to its product suite in conjunction with the HMO products. The CDHP options include Health Savings Accounts (HSAs) and Health Reimbursement Arrangements (HRAs). As with the high-deductible product addition, these features were added in response to changing consumer demands.

Despite management's success in maintaining its high ratings, Healthy Lives has struggled recently given market conditions and limited resources. The health plan is substantially smaller in scale than its major competitors and has faced challenges in the market. Healthy Lives operates in a market that comprises large manufacturers that have been hit hard by the economic recession. These companies, in conjunction with their labor unions, have become more resistant to premium price increases, and while they have traditionally preferred nonprofit managed care companies over the national plans, like UnitedHealthcare and Aetna, they have been more willing to allow new entrants into the market. In addition, in an attempt to control benefit costs, these manufacturers have been seeking low-cost products outside of traditional HMOs such as preferred provider organization (PPO) products with substantial deductibles and co-payments which force the consumer/ employee to bear a larger portion of the costs. These companies have become more price sensitive and increasingly are demanding more low-cost options.

Background

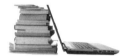

The formation of the health system-owned (provider-owned) health plan was originally undertaken because SMHS saw real value in an integrated approach to the delivery of care that initially could be achieved only by closely linking the payor and provider functions. However, the degree of strategic "fit" has declined. As a provider-owned health plan, Healthy Lives contracts with the hospitals owned by SMHS that operate in its service area. St. Mary's Hospital, the principal SMHS hospital in the health plan's market, has had a problematic relationship with Healthy Lives. The contractual relationship between the hospital and health plan is not accretive on a fully-allocated cost basis to the hospital despite renewed efforts by both parties. The plan has tried to address these losses to the hospital but given its market position it has limited ability. The price sensitivity of clients has pressured the health plan to keep premiums low, which means that it has been unable to raise premiums higher to offer the hospital high enough rates to cover the full healthcare costs of its members. This uneconomical relationship has persisted because Healthy Lives and St. Mary's Hospital are both owned by SMHS, and therefore, the losses are overlooked as transfer pricing issues, not real economic losses. St. Mary's Hospital would not enter into a contract with Healthy Lives at the same rates if the health plan was owned by a third party. In fact, other health plans in the market offer better rates.

Over the last several years, Healthy Lives has had uneven profitability and its premium rates have not kept pace with healthcare costs. It has been unable to grow market share significantly and membership has been declining in the traditional HMO product. Healthy Lives management's strategy for product diversification has been perceived by the SMHS executive leadership team as being too late to the market, given that the health plan will confront substantial competition from larger participants with a broader range of health benefits products. In addition, Healthy Lives will likely face substantial risk in 2014 when employer clients are able to "dump" employees onto the public exchanges under healthcare reform with minimum penalty.

Management undertook a strategic assessment two years ago to identify improvement initiatives. It commenced a turnaround plan to improve financial performance by exiting unprofitable product lines and reducing staff, decreasing administrative expenses, increasing premiums, and implementing a more intensive medical management program. Two years after implementation, however, the health plan fell short of its targets, specifically with respect to premium increases, due largely to market forces out of management's control. Healthy Lives premium increases have historically lagged behind those of larger competitors given its limited leverage in the market, particularly against the large manufacturer customers, and its benefit designs. Management has been more successful in reducing administrative expenses, decreasing the health plan's administrative loss ratio (ALR) from 14% to 11%.

Next Steps

SMHS recently hired a new CEO. As one of his first major initiatives, the CEO decides to undertake an evaluation of Healthy Lives. He soon realizes that Healthy Lives has had mixed financial results over the last five years, and although it has shown some improvement, it is still perceived by St. Mary's Hospital as not paying "fair market" rates. He hires a financial advisor to conduct a strategic options assessment for the health plan, and evaluate the strategic rationale for SMHS to continue to own Healthy Lives. In assessing the strategic options available to Healthy Lives, the financial advisor considers the health plan's current strategic and financial position, and uses the following key evaluation criteria:

- Effect on the market positions of Healthy Lives and St. Mary's Hospital.
- Implications on the relationships among physicians and other ancillary providers in the market and St. Mary's Hospital.
- Mission discernment.
- Effect on the financial positions of Healthy Lives, St. Mary's Hospital, and SMHS.
- Current market value of Healthy Lives and the potential return on investment for SMHS.
- Execution risk and likelihood of success.

After several months of diligence and analysis, the financial advisor presents the following strategic options for Healthy Lives:

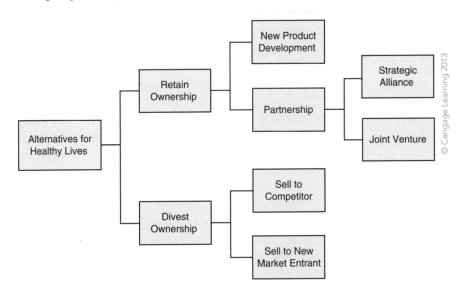

Discussion Questions

1. Discuss each of the strategic options, including a description of the option, the advantages, and the disadvantages. Consider the advantages and disadvantages from the perspective of Healthy Lives, SMHS, and St. Mary's Hospital.

2. How would you assess the best strategic option for Healthy Lives?

3. Discuss why SMHS originally saw value in an integrated approach to the delivery of care that it thought could only be achieved by closely linking the provider and payor functions through ownership of both a hospital and health plan. Do you see any similar trends in the healthcare industry today?

4. In a sale of the health plan, how would you weigh the relative trade-off between the financial value of Healthy Lives as a stand-alone business and the managed care contract terms between Healthy Lives (under new ownership) and St. Mary's Hospital?

5. How might a divestiture of Healthy Lives be the most attractive option for SMHS? For Healthy Lives?

Case 4

The Mission Discernment Process

CASE CONTRIBUTOR Scott D. Musch

Situation

St. Mary's Health System (SMHS) is a nonprofit Catholic healthcare organization. As described in Case 3, the new CEO recently hired a financial advisor to conduct a strategic options assessment for SMHS's health plan, Healthy Lives. The SMHS executive leadership team is in the process of weighing the options against different criteria, which include preserving the payor/provider relationship, improving its market position, improving its financial position, maximizing the valuation of Healthy Lives, maximizing its return on investment in the health plan, successfully executing a transaction, and meeting mission discernment. The last objective—meet mission discernment—involves a detailed process for the executive leadership team. Like other faith-based, nonprofit organizations, SMHS measures its accomplishments as an organization in terms of its success in realizing its mission and values.

Background

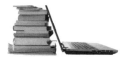

Faith-based healthcare organizations use the mission discernment process to ensure that in the course of making major decisions it uses appropriate business and clinical analyses guided by its mission and core values. For instance, these major decisions might include a merger, acquisition, or business partnership; significant capital expenditures; or major service line expansions or reductions. As an example, one Catholic health system uses the mission discernment process whenever it is confronted with a significant decision that:

- might alter or appear to affect the Catholic identity of the organization;
- might positively or negatively impact the mission of the organization;
- might significantly affect the status of groups of employees; or
- might affect local communities, vulnerable populations, or the environment.

As part of the process, Catholic health systems consider if such decisions will be consistent with the published *Ethical and Religious Directives for Catholic Health Care Services* (ERDs). The ERDs are outlined in a document that offers moral guidance and ethical direction on various aspects of healthcare delivery.

The mission discernment process is the responsibility of the executives who will be making the decision. As soon as a major initiative is underway, senior leaders will establish a committee to engage in the process. Members of the committee will analyze the situation, using all available data and pertinent information to identify issues that will need to be resolved or mitigated in order to be consistent with the organization's mission and core values. The committee will prepare a written report that addresses these issues. The report is presented to the executive leadership team or the organization's board of directors. The report does not provide a recommendation but rather serves as support for decision makers to reach a fully-informed decision. The purpose of the mission discernment process is to achieve integration of the mission, business, and clinical elements of a proposed initiative.

Next Steps

The SMHS executive team formed a committee to engage in the mission discernment process for consideration of the preferred strategic option for the health plan. The committee is considering the following strategic options for the health plan:

- Retain ownership and launch new products.
- Partner through a strategic alliance.
- Partner through a joint venture.
- Sell 100% of the health plan to an in-market competitor.
- Sell 100% of the health plan to a new market entrant.

The committee is tasked with identifying and reporting how each option relates to the organization's mission and core values.

Discussion Questions

1. How might the decision to pursue a strategic transaction for Healthy Lives affect the organization's mission?

2. Identify reasons for or against each strategic option as it relates to its ability to help SMHS realize its mission as a Catholic health system (refer to the *Ethical and Religious Directives for Catholic Health Care Services*, Fourth Edition, http://old .usccb.org/bishops/directives.shtml#partone).

3. Who from Healthy Lives should be on the committee?

4. How does the mission discernment process help a healthcare organization maintain adherence to its mission and core values?

5. How might the mission discernment process conflict with the turnaround strategy of a health plan that is financially struggling?

Case 5

Rural Healthcare Development under Healthcare Reform

CASE CONTRIBUTOR **Steve Barnett**

Situation

Landen Cook and Braedyn Brewer are the CEOs of neighboring Critical Access Hospitals (CAHs) in Sanilac County, Michigan. Since 2008, both CAHs have experienced declining patient revenue, rising unemployment, and increasing bad debt. In 2010, recognizing the need to establish a cooperative relationship, Landen and Braedyn began discussing the future of health care in light of the recently enacted Patient Protection and Affordable Care Act (PPACA). The conversation progressed to the point of committing to work collaboratively and to explore shared service opportunities beginning in 2011. While identifying shared service opportunities, Landen and Braedyn both recognized that healthcare systems in adjacent counties were increasingly interested in their shared populations. This, coupled with their intent to assess the possibility of forming an accountable care organization (ACO), led them to the realization that merging their two facilities might be beneficial. Merging the two CAHs and forming an ACO also has led Landen and Braedyn to realize that they will need a tertiary hospital partner.

Both CAHs are nonprofit organizations. Landen's CAH is structured under a corporate holding company, while Braedyn's CAH has a large board of incorporators. A board of incorporators is a large community membership (30–50 people) that meets once a year for a progress report on a hospital. The board of incorporators selects the hospital board (8–10 people) and votes on issues such as mergers. This board structure is a relatively old form and in many cases adds a layer of complexity in gaining approval. Braedyn's board of incorporators is not particularly well informed about matters of health care, and yet must approve the merger. Although both CAHs have a formal patient transfer relationship with the same large independent community hospital, neither has a formal transfer relationship with a tertiary facility. The surrounding adjacent counties have four evolving healthcare systems of which three have a tertiary facility in their system. Landen and Braedyn have analyzed their combined patient out-migration traffic and discovered that no pattern exists. According to 2010 census data, there were 39,617 people in their combined primary and secondary service areas, with a projected 3% decline by 2015. Currently, their combined unique total patients being seen by their primary care providers is 19,294, of which 45% are Medicare beneficiaries. This patient population is expected to grow 4% by 2015.

Background

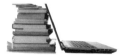

In March 2010, the most significant opportunity to change how health care is delivered in the United States was enacted through the enactment of the PPACA. Embedded in PPACA is a new delivery and payment model called an accountable care organization. An ACO can apply for traditional fee-for-service Medicare patients in its geographical location. The benefit to the ACO model is that the participants will share in the savings related to the past three years' healthcare services utilization of those Medicare beneficiaries assigned to it. The ACO is obligated to manage all the healthcare needs of a Medicare patient population of not less than 5000, which may require services that fall outside the scope of care offered by the ACO. Although the payment system is a mix of fee-for-service and shared savings, the opportunity represents a shift toward population health management.

Rural health care is typically provided by small hospitals with fewer than 50 staffed beds. In many cases, these small hospitals have converted to a CAH designation, which provides for cost-based reimbursement from Medicare. The CAH program has been popular even though there are some restrictions, one of which is a maximum of 25 staffed beds. Small rural hospitals are important local economic drivers as they employ many of the physicians in a community and own the ambulance, home care, and other affiliated healthcare services. These rural facilities have transfer relationships with larger hospitals, although those larger hospitals may not always be tertiary facilities. Most of the rural CAHs are independent nonprofit organizations that historically have competed with neighboring facilities and are not accustomed to working collaboratively.

Next Steps

Landen and Braedyn are clearly concerned about the future of rural health care and their ability to remain as independent hospitals. Both organizations are financially struggling and this is directly related to the economic crisis and its impact on a historically industrial environment in the community. They are also working aggressively to incorporate programs related to electronic health records and quality care measures that will impact how they are paid in the near term. Both organizations understand the need to work collaboratively. They realize the potential need to merge and acknowledge that if they are to develop an ACO, they will need a tertiary hospital that fulfills their unmet service needs. Landen and Braedyn are preparing to present their strategic vision to their respective boards. They believe their strategy will preserve healthcare services for their communities in the future. However, they face a number of challenges, one of which is how to decide what tertiary hospital would be a good partner.

Discussion Questions

1. Describe Landen and Braedyn's shared vision for their CAHs.

2. Given the independent and historical competitive relationship between the CAHs, what cultural changes do you think need to be assessed and/or considered?

3. What problems may Landen and Braedyn encounter when they propose a merger to their larger communities, and in particular, Braedyn's board of incorporators?

4. What is the benefit of forming an ACO? What issues do Landen and Braedyn need to consider in forming an ACO?

5. Does the census data in the scenario and combined Medicare volume support the ACO criteria for beneficiary qualification?

6. If Landen and Braedyn want to retain control over how health care is delivered in their communities, how should they manage the selection of a tertiary facility in the potential merger?

7. What role should a tertiary partner have in a proposed rural healthcare system?

Case 6

A Change in Culture at a CCRC

CASE CONTRIBUTOR **Matthew Bogner**

Situation

A historic continuing care retirement community with a rich and proud heritage is forced to reposition due to changing consumer preferences and market demand. New leadership advocates for culture change in aging services, moving away from the hospital-based institutional model of care to the "household model" that advocates for the creation of a true home both architecturally and internally. The leadership team contracts with national consultants to assist with deep-seated internal change while at the same time planning a $22 million household renovation that will affect each area of campus.

Background

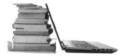

Kansas Masonic Home is a beautiful mission-style retirement community in Wichita, Kansas. Founded in 1896 to serve "the aged, infirm, widows and orphans," the organization has repositioned several times over the years to meet the changing needs of the fraternity and community. During this time, Kansas Masonic Home has met many challenges. Early in the history of the organization, a devastating fire took the lives of five residents and destroyed the original campus. However, the legacy of care survived. The organization quickly rebuilt and withstood two world wars and a whole host of other challenges over the years. A brief timeline of the organization highlights other major operational changes. In 1959, for the first time in 60 years there was not one child in residence. Senior care became the greatest need and focus of operations. In 1986, Kansas Masonic Home opened to the public. For the first time in 90 years, Masonic or Eastern Star heritage or membership was not required for residency. In 1994, the independent living Towers opened on the west side of campus. In 1998, the assisted living Manor opened and the campus officially became a continuing care retirement community (CCRC). Many important strategic decisions were made throughout the organization's history and it flourished under leadership's vision and ability to change. However, by 2008 the organization was struggling. Instability in senior leadership and an institutional mindset had limited innovation and growth in the organization. Consumer preferences had also begun to change. In addition, competition increased in the local market. The organization found that census was on the decline and a dramatic repositioning was needed to remain a vibrant and financially solid organization.

Next Steps

A new administrator was hired at this time and was subsequently promoted to CEO. He knew the organization needed to change from "institution" to "home." This change was evident by the lack of choice residents exhibited over their daily lives and the way care was being provided. The CEO also felt the best way to do this was by providing care in small households with permanent, small, care teams. As he shared this vision with the board of directors and leadership team, there was a consensus that none of them wanted to live the rest of their lives in a hospital. But this was exactly what they were providing! The CEO understood the first step to change was a deep understanding of the organization's strengths, weaknesses, market demand, and competition. The leadership team therefore requested a marketing study from a regional consultant. The study showed that the independent living units were too small to be competitive, but would be acceptable as assisted living units. The current assisted living units were too small as well, but would be acceptable for memory care assisted living. Finally, the healthcare units were mostly semiprivate while consumers were demanding private rooms. Like most traditional "nursing homes," the healthcare center also looked more like a hospital than a home. Therefore, the leadership team developed a plan to convert independent living into assisted living units, assisted living into three households including two memory care households, and the healthcare center into four 20-bed households with predominately private rooms. They also found there was demand for a state-of-the-art 20-bed rehabilitation household for short-stay residents. Over the next few years, they completed the design, development, and financing of the project. They also worked with national consultants to assist with staff training, blending of roles, restructuring of decision making processes, and systems with the intent of "making it home."

Discussion Questions

1. How would you educate staff, residents, and families about this paradigm shift?

2. How would interdisciplinary decision making play a role in the change process?

3. How would a goal of 100% stakeholder involvement benefit the change process?

4. What would you want your life to be like if you needed this type of care?

5. Has a family member ever needed long-term care? How was that experience?

Group Exercise

Hand out a blank sheet of paper and a pencil to each participant. Ask them to privately write down answers to the following questions:

    If you were a resident in a "nursing home":

- What time would you get up?
- What would you eat for breakfast?
- What activities would you like to do?

- When/how often would you bathe?
- What time would you go to bed?

When participants are done, ask them to pass their paper to the person on their right. Now ask participants to study this new piece of paper and the preferences in front of them. Ask: "What if this were your schedule from now on . . . is there anything that would bother you?" Use this as a basis for discussing the lack of choice traditional nursing homes afford the residents who live there. Discuss "culture change" in aging services.

Case 7

Addressing the Psychological Effects of Exposure to Community Violence

CASE CONTRIBUTOR **Frank J. Corigliano**

Situation

Dr. Alexander Davidson, chief of community care at the James County Medical Center, reviewed the reports on his desk, which documented the high rates of exposure to community violence in his catchment area. He was particularly concerned because he knew that exposure to community violence is associated with serious emotional and behavioral problems. As the chief of community care, he was troubled by the number of patients who present with serious psychological problems but are not properly identified or effectively treated. Dr. Davidson believes that many of the presenting problems of his patients such as hypertension, obesity, and somatic complaints could also be effectively treated with the integration of psychological care throughout the medical center.

Although there is little that Dr. Davidson can do directly to change the levels of exposure to violence in the community, he believes that there is much that can be done when these individuals enter the walls of the medical center. How can Dr. Davidson achieve the goals of identifying and caring for the physical and mental health of the patients in his community? Dr. Davidson is aware that there is sometimes a stigma related to mental health treatment. He is concerned that many of his patients, staff, and administrators may not be well informed about the important role of psychology in a medical setting. Dr. Davidson is committed to developing a policy that harnesses the unique resources of his organization to effect change in his community.

Background

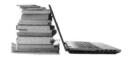

Millions of Americans reside in communities with high rates of interpersonal violence. A recent report indicated that in 2009, in New York City alone, there were 46,357 violent crimes, including 471 murders, 832 forcible rapes, 18,597 robberies, and 26,457 aggravated assaults.[1] These residents are at increased risk for exposure to community violence. Community violence is defined as serious interpersonal violence (such as being chased, beaten up, shot or shot at, raped, or attacked with a weapon) that occurs outside the home. Often distinctions are made between primary, secondary, and tertiary exposure (victim, witness, or even just hearing about a violent act in the community). Exposure to community violence presents as a critical public health problem as each of these exposures is associated with serious negative effects on psychological well-being. Exposure to community violence continues to be associated with unwanted psychological correlates and emotional and behavioral problems such as depression, anxiety, and aggression, and significantly affects the lives of the individuals living in these communities.[2]

Individuals who experience untreated psychological challenges, such as depression and anxiety, tend to have more frequent hospital visits and require greater levels of medical care. Often seeking treatment for physical care is more acceptable than for mental health. For example, it has been suggested that up to 75% of primary care visits are associated with problems that respond well to psychological interventions such as emotional and behavioral correlates such as hypertension, diabetes, nutrition, exercise, cancer, depression, and anxiety. Community programs such as university-administered psychological centers or school-based violence de-escalation programs work from within the communities they serve to provide support and treatment of problems like anxiety, depression, and aggression that can be related to exposure to violence.

The Centers for Disease Control and Prevention (CDC) has long recognized community violence as a key public health priority that can have serious implications on public health. In 1979, the U.S. Surgeon General identified violent behavior as a key public health priority. In 1980, the CDC began studying patterns of violence and developed a national program to reduce the death and disability associated with injuries outside the workplace. In 1992, the CDC established the National Center for Injury Prevention and Control (NCIPC) as the lead federal organization for violence prevention. Within the NCIPC, the Division of Violence Prevention (DVP) works to prevent injuries and deaths caused by violence (see www.cdc.gov/ViolencePrevention/overview/index.html). The CDC has recommended a public health approach through a four-step process that can be applied to violence and other health problems that affect populations: (1) Define the problem; (2) Identify risk and protective factors; (3) Develop and test prevention strategies; and (4) Assure widespread adoption.[3]

Next Steps

To respond to the problem, Dr. Davidson developed patient and community outreach programs that emphasize education and positive results to convince patients, staff, and administrators of the gap in care related to mental health. Dr. Davidson has investigated available public health resources to help accomplish these goals. He recognized that some people are concerned about possible stigma of mental illness. He also understands that especially in some cultures, depression and anxiety are perceived as signs of weakness, a perception that is not favored in these tough inner-city communities. However, his message is that strength comes from supporting individuals' mental health and serving the community as a whole. By intervening at the individual level in the medical center setting, individuals who are exposed to violence might receive the treatment that may reduce the risk of becoming a victim, and thus reduce the risk of becoming an offender. Dr. Davidson hopes that intervening to support mental health at the hospital level by identifying and treating individuals with psychological service needs may serve to break the cycle of violence in the community.

Discussion Questions

1. How can Dr. Davidson work with public health agencies—both government and volunteer, non-profit organizations—to achieve his goals?

2. Given the high rates of community violence in Dr. Davidson's catchment area, what strategies would you recommend to Dr. Davidson to integrate psychological care into the physical healthcare environments, such as hospitals, medical centers, and other healthcare organizations?

3. How can public health organizations support hospital administrators and physicians to identify and engage patients who could likely benefit from psychological treatment but face challenges in access, lack of awareness, and refusal to acknowledge mental health needs?

4. As a public health official, how do you promote the integration of psychological health into hospitals as a civil responsibility?

5. How can public health organizations work with professional groups, such as primary care and mental health doctors, to be instrumental in changing the stigma associated with mental health illness, particularly as related to inner-city communities?

6. In what ways can public health agencies support communities that are affected by high rates of community violence and the correlated negative impact on physical and mental health?

References

1 Federal Bureau of Investigation, U.S. Department of Justice. (2010, September). Offences known to law enforcement by metropolitan statistical area, 2009 [Table 6]. *Crime in the United States, 2009.* Retrieved from http://www.fbi.gov/about-us/cjis/ucr/crime-in-the-u.s/2009

2 Corigliano, F. J. (2011). *Community violence exposure and behavioral and emotional functioning among African American and Latino children and adolescents: A nonpsychiatric inpatient sample* (Unpublished doctoral dissertation). St. John's University, New York.

3 Centers for Disease Control and Prevention (CDC). (2008, March 5). *Violence prevention.* Retrieved from the CDC, Injury Center at http://www.cdc.gov/ncipc/dvp/PublicHealthApproachTo_ViolencePrevention.htm

Case 8

CASE CONTRIBUTOR **Stanley A. Phillip, Jr.**

Situation

Dr. Denise Ellington, program lead, was tapped to lead the newly created Community Based Organization (CBO)/Health Department Program Operation Team (CHPOT) within the Division of HIV/AIDS Prevention (DHAP), Prevention Program Branch (PPB) of the Centers for Disease Control and Prevention (CDC). She enthusiastically embraced her new role and was particularly excited at the prospect of leading a team that is charged with developing the new program announcement for the soon-to-end Expanded Testing Initiative. In preparation for what Dr. Ellington considered her most challenging career effort, she pored over the myriad of reports and data collected during the past three years for the first initiative. She quickly realized that even though the program achieved many milestones against the original objectives, the new announcement must incorporate lessons learned to mitigate potential challenges and barriers that stymied programmatic implementation of the Expanded Testing Initiative.

Background

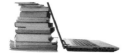

In 2007, the CDC funded the program announcement *PS07-768 Expanded and Integrated Human Immunodeficiency Virus (HIV) Testing for Populations Disproportionately Affected by HIV, Primarily African Americans*, a three-year program to expand testing in clinical and nonclinical settings. The goals of the Expanded Testing Initiative were to conduct 1.5 million tests and identify 20,000 newly reported cases of HIV infection annually; at least 80% of funding must support HIV testing in healthcare (clinical) settings and up to 20% of funding could support testing in non-healthcare (community-based) settings. The initiative capitalized on an existing healthcare workforce and service delivery that had the requisite personnel, expertise, and infrastructure to effectively and efficiently carry out activities that supported the testing initiative. The only aspect of the initiative that was new or fairly unchartered was the introduction of routine HIV testing in clinical settings. This intersection of prevention and care proved to be a major barrier to the realization of the central thrust of the initiative, routine HIV testing in a clinical setting. While Year 1 was beset with startup challenges and unanticipated barriers, including confusion about establishing reasonable objectives, Year 2 was marked with significant improvement. Funded programs addressed most of the challenges experienced in Year 1 and dramatically improved their success with the implementation of the program, reaching their goals and objectives.

The Expanded Testing Initiative is part of a comprehensive response to heighten awareness of the disproportionate burden the HIV/AIDS epidemic has on the African American community. Leadership and governance, as well as health financing, were multilayered in the sense that Congress authorized the funding ($35 million) and the Department of Health and Human Services via the PPB developed the policy framework for the funding opportunity announcement (FOA). The FOA is the financial vehicle by which the public may access public funds to support programs in local jurisdictions.

As is true with the implementation of any new initiative, the funded programs faced many barriers and challenges to reach the stated goals. During implementation there were some noted barriers:

- Legislative: HIV policies and informed consent;
- Start-up: obtaining buy-in from healthcare settings (e.g., emergency departments), establishing contracts, establishing new protocols and structures, getting new resources;
- Financial: budget cuts and obtaining reimbursement;
- Operational: HIV testing saturation, repeat testing, testing space, natural disasters, and stigma and patients' resistance;
- Staffing: resistance to change, overburdened staff, and state hiring freezes;
- Data collection and reporting: data flow, data integration of testing into existing data bases, data entry backlog, incomplete data forms, and nonstandardized data reporting burden associated with data collection and reporting; and
- Barriers specific to program sites (e.g., correctional settings: low positivity rates, funding, security issues, and buy-in).

Next Steps

Dr. Ellington has the responsibility to lead the CHPOT to develop the new FOA which will replace the existing Expanded Testing Initiative for the next three years (2010–2013). The PPB staffs and project officers actively manage and support HIV prevention activities in 50 states, the District of Columbia, Puerto Rico, the U.S. Virgin Islands, and Affiliated Pacific Island jurisdictions. Many jurisdictions' HIV prevention programs are often supported via multiple funding streams (i.e., FOA) and Dr. Ellington must ensure HIV prevention efforts are comprehensive, capitalizing on synergies and limiting or removing barriers to prevention efforts.

To develop an FOA, Dr. Ellington must coordinate the CHPOT to review and analyze the outcome of the Expanded Testing Initiative taking into consideration the following:

- Promotion of integrated testing activities, avoidance of stand-alone or parallel testing programs;
- Provision of guidance and support to jurisdictions that have legislation in place that may present challenges to full integration of HIV prevention testing activities; and
- Ensure that funded activities result in an overall increase of jurisdictional HIV testing.

Discussion Questions

1. Understanding the need to develop a new FOA that takes into consideration past challenges, who should Dr. Ellington and the CHPOT consult?

2. What method should the CHPOT employ to obtain this feedback?

3. How can the team encourage and facilitate coordination and collaboration of stakeholders in the varied jurisdictions?

4. Should funding levels be tied to implementation success, documented need, or a combination of both?

5. What are some of the challenges Dr. Ellington and the CHPOT will face in incorporating lessons learned from the past into the new program?

Case 9

Dropping Small-Group Insurance Products

CASE CONTRIBUTOR Scott D. Musch

Situation

A large, publicly-traded national health insurance company, GreenHealth, announced its decision to drop a number of small-group insurance products in Virginia because of financial losses. Originally scheduled to occur in four months, GreenHealth has agreed to allow customers affected by the decision to continue on their existing products until their scheduled renewal dates, at which point the products will be stopped. The company will continue to offer a number of small-group products in the state, although the remaining product options will generally have higher premiums and less attractive benefits.

Paul Dennis, VP of Small Group Products for GreenHealth, advocated for the decision to drop the products instead of proposing a rate increase, which would have required GreenHealth to justify the increase to the state. The change will have a significant impact on the company's small-group product line in Virginia and will result in lower risk membership and lower revenues through reduced premiums, but also higher earnings. The small-group market for GreenHealth has been losing money for the company for the last two years. The products being dropped are the ones that have the most consumer demand, including the company's most popular health insurance plan, WorkHealth EPO (exclusive provider organization). The products that will be retained are much less cost competitive in the market. Small employers in Virginia do not have many plans left from which to choose. GreenHealth originally planned a hard stop of the products in four months, however, the insurance regulators pushed back and GreenHealth compromised with allowing the coverages to end on renewal dates. The regulators had an issue with ending the coverages abruptly as it would have affected customers' deductibles and out-of-pocket maximums.

Paul, in defending the company's decision to regulators and consumer advocates, argued that the small-group market in the state has been dysfunctional for a long time. The primary issues include community rating for premium rates (meaning everyone pays the same price), guaranteed issue (meaning health plans cannot turn individuals or groups down, regardless of preexisting conditions), and no requirement that anyone within a market buy insurance. Paul specifically cited adverse selection, hospital rate increases, and low premiums for mandated products as reasons. Recently it has become very difficult for health plans to obtain rate increases. Virginia is one of a number of states that has authority to deny proposed premium increases and under the Patient Protection and Affordable Care Act (PPACA), the Centers for Medicare & Medicaid Services (CMS) now has authority in conjunction with states to review potentially unreasonable increases in health insurance premiums to determine whether rate increases are justified. Under PPACA, CMS can provide states with supplemental funding to strengthen a state's rate review process.

Background

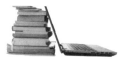

According to America's Health Insurance Plans (AHIP) organization, small groups are classified as companies with 2 to 50 employees. Insurance coverage for small groups generally is fully insured. Employers purchase an insurance contract from a licensed health insurer or HMO, which assumes the full financial risk for paying healthcare claims. Small-group health insurance is offered on a guarantee-issue basis, meaning a small business cannot be denied coverage due to the health status or illness of its employees or their dependents. A majority of states have adopted premium rating rules that place limits on rate adjustments, including for such factors as health status and claims experience of the enrollees of a group.

Next Steps

GreenHealth has approximately 300,000 small-group members in Virginia. Paul anticipates that the company only risks losing one-third of those covered lives since he expects many of the affected employers will switch to one of the higher cost products that GreenHealth will continue to offer. Small employers in Virginia do not have many other plans from which to choose. In general, small employer-sponsored insurance coverage will undergo significant changes under PPACA starting in 2014 when the health insurance exchanges are in place. Paul recognizes that given the significantly higher premiums and lower benefits offered by the products that remain, the company's membership losses could be much larger than anticipated. In 2011, with the 300,000 small-group covered lives, GreenHealth earned $1.4 billion in premiums but reported a medical loss ratio of 89.5%. The company's administrative expense ratio in Virginia hovered around 12.8%, generating a negative operating margin of 2.3%. Assuming a loss of 100,000 covered lives, Paul estimates the small-group product line in Virginia will swing to a positive operating margin (see Table 9–1) despite the negative fixed administrative leverage that the company would experience from losing nearly $600 million in premiums.

Table 9–1 GreenHealth's Small-Group Product Financials in Virginia (2011)

	2011		Pro Forma	
		PMPM*		PMPM*
Covered Lives	300,000		200,000	
Member Months	3,060,000		2,040,000	
Premiums	$1,400,000,000	$388.89	$836,502,000	$410.05
Medical Expenses	$1,253,000,000	$348.06	$714,000,000	$350.00
Medical Loss Ratio (MLR)	89.5%		85.4%	
Medical Margin	$147,000,000	$40.83	$122,502,000	$60.05
Administrative Expenses	$178,500,000	$49.58	$112,927,770	$55.36
Administrative Expense Ratio	12.8%		13.50%	
Operating Profit	($31,500,000)	($8.75)	$9,574,230	$4.69
Operating Profit Margin	–2.3%	–2.3%	1.1%	1.1%

*Per member per month

Discussion Questions

1. Review Table 9–1 and discuss the implications of losing 100,000 covered lives by targeting the elimination by GreenHealth of specific small-group products.

2. GreenHealth's small-group business in Virginia has a certain level of fixed administrative expenses that it must maintain for operations in the state. What are the risks if more employers than expected do not switch into one of the company's higher cost products?

3. Discuss what factors a health insurance company should consider in deciding whether to drop an unprofitable product or increase premium rates given the potential negative effects on customers.

4. What factors should be considered by state regulators in determining if an increase in insurance premium rates is unreasonable?

5. Are state rate review processes, strengthen by PPACA, a victory for consumers if it ultimately means that health insurance companies drop products that become unprofitable?

6. Research the effects of PPACA on small businesses and their workers.

Case 10 — Managing Retail-Based Health Clinics: Financial Performance and Mission

CASE CONTRIBUTORS Patrick M. Hermanson and Tracy J. Farnsworth

Situation

Jeanne Wagner faced a professional challenge when she was told the retail-based health clinic she was responsible for had to break even or be closed by year-end. Jeanne began working for American Health Systems (AHS), a national chain of for-profit hospitals, when her hospital, Pleasant Valley Medical Center (PVMC), was acquired by AHS in 2008. Historically, PVMC's mission was to provide cost-effective, quality health care to everyone regardless of the ability to pay. With new owners and a heightened focus on profits, every PVMC service had to demonstrate a financial contribution to the organization's success—and Jeanne's retail-based health clinic required significant changes to survive.

Jeanne accepted employment at PVMC because she wanted to help people. She liked healthcare management and received her master's degree in Health Administration. Eventually, Jeanne was promoted and placed in charge of all ambulatory care clinics at PVMC. Over the years she was given additional responsibilities and was thrilled when asked to open a retail-based health clinic to meet an important and previously unmet community need.

Background

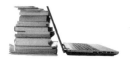

Jeanne was already a key player for PVMC when it decided to go into retail-based health care. Prior to the hospital's sale, PVMC had completed a community needs assessment and learned that access to care was a significant issue in Pleasant Valley. The uninsured in general and lower income families in particular were often denied needed patient care because they lacked access to a convenient, cost-effective alternative to a physician office, urgent care, or hospital emergency room.

Upon researching the market, Jeanne learned about the relatively recent phenomenon of retail-based health clinics and in her travels observed several clinics located in "big box" retail outlets such as Target, Walmart, CVS Pharmacy, and Kroger grocery stores. Jeanne knew that the development of a retail-based health clinic in Pleasant Valley might threaten local physicians; however, it would be an opportunity to expand access to care to the entire population. She also knew that if PVMC was not the first to market with this new innovation, it would likely be done by a competitor.

During that same period, PVMC was becoming increasingly concerned about the predatory marketing activities being conducted in their community by Freedom Health-care (FH), a rival institution less than 30 miles away. FH recently acquired land for a hospital-sponsored medical group office building and continually ran radio and television advertisements recommending patients travel to their community for care. FH also placed several billboards and newspaper ads that subtly criticized the perceived weaknesses of PVMC. Thus, development of a defensive strategy became a primary focus of PVMC's hospital administration and board of directors, and the development of retail-based health clinics became a key component of PVMV's amended strategic plan.

Immediately after gaining approval to develop a retail-based health clinic, Jeanne identified a local retailer that wanted to partner with PVMC to open a clinic. She attended an orientation at the retailer's headquarters, negotiated a detailed lease agreement, and be-gan to recruit the needed staff to open the clinic. The first three years after Jeanne opened the clinic it performed as expected—it lost money based on limited patient visits. Of course clinic volume was expected to grow as word got out and the community grew comfortable with retail-based healthcare delivery.

As Jeanne reflected upon the clinic's limited volume and significant financial loss, she understood that several factors were prohibiting her success, including marketing limita-tions built into the lease that made it extremely difficult to create awareness and familiarity within the target population. In addition, the clinic's location within the store was neither visually nor practically optimal for initiating patient care. In addition, Jeanne was never able to directly employ the providers in the clinic, but was forced for political reasons to contract with a local primary care provider who provided the advanced practice profession-als (APPs). This arrangement added cost without any added value.

Next Steps

When PVMC was sold to AHS, a new strategic plan was developed that reflected a sig-nificant change in direction from the previous plan. Since AHS is a for-profit healthcare company, it must provide a return to investors, thus the expectations for earnings before interest, taxes, depreciation, and amortization (EBITDA) was more than doubled from pre-vious targets. PVMC still provided a reasonable amount of indigent care, but it necessar-ily was much more focused on financial metrics. Service line managers like Jeanne were expected to make the changes necessary to bring their services to profitability. Jeanne was asked to turn the retail-based health clinic around by end of the fiscal year or risk being closed. In summary, she was faced with two difficult issues. First, how could she continue to meet the community needs for cost-effective, convenient care if her clinic was closed? And second, what must be done to make her clinic profitable?

Discussion Questions

1. What immediate, intermediate, and long-term steps should Jeanne take to turn her retail-based health clinic around financially?

2. What could have been done in the planning phase to ensure success of the retail-based health clinic?

3. What data, resources, and support does Jeanne need in order to address the expectations of her administration?

4. How can Jeanne meet her ethical commitment to provide care to everyone regardless of the ability to pay and still meet the obligation to shareholders for a return on investment?

Case 11 — Rural Medical Practice—Balancing Needs and Necessities

CASE CONTRIBUTOR James Allen Johnson, III

Situation

Dr. Marvin Whitson is the physician and owner of a private primary care medical practice in Lake Sophia, Florida. The medical practice serves approximately 500 active patients and operates as a family practice providing primary care services to all age groups. Like many medical practices, most patients are elderly and have Medicare benefits.

Carson Johnson was recently hired as chief administrator of the medical practice. He discovered that approximately 25% of their patients have outstanding balances, some of which have accumulated over the course of several years. After further investigation, Carson realized that many of the debts are as high as several thousand dollars. The medical practice's balance sheets indicate that for the past five years the practice barely breaks even each year. He confirmed that if the practice were to maintain as it has been, it would be losing money within two years.

Background

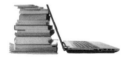

Lake Sophia is a small town with approximately 2,000 residents located in a rural area of central Florida. The town of Lake Sophia is located in one of the poorest areas in the state. The health of the population of Lake Sophia reflects its socioeconomic status (SES) in that, not only does it have some of the lowest SES indicators (income, education, and occupation) in Florida, but its population has some of the worst health as well.

Concerned with his findings, Carson confronted Dr. Whitson about the situation. The doctor informed Carson that he was aware of the problem and that he wanted it to be addressed somehow but was concerned that because many of his patients had low incomes or were impoverished, measures employed to correct the problem could have a tremendous impact on the lives of many of these patients. Furthermore, Dr. Whitson once tried to gain insight into the problem and found that paying the co-payments proved to be a great burden for these patients and they were simply unable to pay. Dr. Whitson was one of only two physicians practicing in Lake Sophia, and felt an obligation to the community to provide medical services to people who needed it. He is also aware that his practice was currently unsustainable and that something must be done; however, it is important that his mission to serve this community not be compromised. The overhead cost at the practice had already been reduced to the bare minimum; furthermore, the practice is at over capacity and is not likely to be able to handle many more patients.

Next Steps

Carson realized he must find a balance between the fiscal and monetary needs of the medical practice and the obligation Dr. Whitson has to his patients and the community. He must account for the realities faced by the population the practice serves while devising a strategic plan that addresses the sustainability of the practice and ensures its longevity.

Discussion Questions

1. What other considerations in regard to the patients who have accumulated debt should Carson account for?

2. What are some ways that revenues could be increased while still adhering to Dr. Whitson's mission?

3. Devise a strategic plan for the practice for the next five years that would address the aforementioned problems.

Case 12

How Do You End an Unprofitable Business Relationship?

CASE CONTRIBUTOR **James A. Johnson**

Situation

Northbridge Rehabilitation Center (Northbridge) opened in December three years ago.[1] The building in which it is housed was purchased from a group of Northbridge businessmen who had hopes of opening the new building as a skilled nursing facility. These businessmen had already hired their clinical managers and contracted a local physician-owned physical therapy group, Pioneer Physical Rehab Inc. (Pioneer), to provide physical therapy services. When Northbridge bought the building, they extended employment opportunities to the clinical managers and signed an agreement to contract physical therapy services from Pioneer. Northbridge admitted patients immediately.

Background

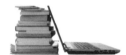

The advantages of retaining the physical therapy contract appeared obvious:

- The therapists were already on board.
- The owner of Pioneer, Dr. Trison, was a prominent orthopedic surgeon in town. By using his physical therapists, Northbridge was almost guaranteed referrals from him.
- Pioneer owned equipment, which decreased the amount of capital expenditures required by Northbridge.

Initially, the agreement worked well. Dr. Trison greatly assisted with filling the rehabilitation beds. He openly supported Northbridge, which helped the facility gain support from other physicians.

Within a year, however, the drawbacks of the contract also became evident:

- Northbridge had no input into the hiring or supervision of the therapists. Although some therapists were excellent, others were less acceptable.
- There were not enough physical therapists sent to Northbridge, and Pioneer was not aggressive in recruiting additional staff.
- The physical therapists were the only clinicians not employed by Northbridge. Their loyalty was mixed and therefore broke down the multidisciplinary approach.
- Good therapists were transferred from Northbridge as Dr. Trison obtained new contracts. These therapists were not always replaced.

- Dr. Trison lost battles with Northbridge about reimbursement, so he began referring much of his outpatient business elsewhere.
- Northbridge physical therapy profits were not maximized by using a contract service.

Next Steps

After three years of operation, Northbridge had developed a good reputation; the beds were full and business was promising in all areas. However, Northbridge considered the physical therapy contract an issue. Dr. Trison made it clear that he was not happy about the possibility of ending the contract. Northbridge knew it would not be a friendly termination. Would the advantages of employing their own physical therapists outweigh the disadvantages? The advantages included increased physical therapy profits; complete control of recruitment, hiring, and supervising of physical therapists; increased Northbridge visibility with respect from the physical therapy professionals in the area; and a strengthened multidisciplinary team approach. On the other hand, they would lose Dr. Trison's support and referrals. They ran the risk that Dr. Trison might develop another form of competition for the clinic, and they would incur the cost of replacing the majority of the physical therapy equipment, which was currently owned by Dr. Trison's group.

Discussion Questions

1. What are the major issues involved?

2. What would your decision be on continuing the contract with Pioneer if you were the Northbridge manager?

3. What would your response be if you were Dr. Trison?

4. What are the probable outcomes of this scenario?

5. Discuss how Northbridge could have improved the contract with Pioneer at inception.

Reference

[1] Kilpatrick, A. O., & Johnson, J. A. (1999). *Human resources and organizational behavior: Cases in health services management*. Chicago: Health Administration Press.

Case 13 — Budget Cuts in a Home Care Program

CASE CONTRIBUTOR Scott D. Musch

Situation

Pauline, a director of the California Department of Social Services (CDSS) for San Martin County, returned to her office after a meeting with the County Board of Supervisors. The board of supervisors was considering drastic reductions in the proposed funding for the county's In-Home Supportive Services (IHSS) program. Similar to most municipalities in California, San Martin County faced a substantial budget deficit in the upcoming fiscal year. The economic downturn coupled with the state's budget problems had a lingering effect on the county's revenues. The county relied on matching state funds to support the IHSS program. Given the state's fiscal woes, the governor was likely to propose significant cuts in all social programs, including IHSS, to try to stop some of the fiscal bleeding. In fact, the previous governor in his last year of office had proposed cutting roughly half the funding for the IHSS program. Therefore, it was unlikely that the county would escape funding cuts from the state and it had to make some drastic decisions.

The board of supervisors tasked Pauline with working with San Martin County's IHSS Public Authority Governing Board to come up with some budget recommendations. Primary among those recommendations will be significant cuts in the wages and benefits of the home care workers for the IHSS program. Pauline knows that entertaining such discussions will ignite a backlash from the Service Employees International Union—United Healthcare Workers West (SEIU), which represents the county's home care workers. The county's collective bargaining contract with the Local SEIU expires in two months and the board of supervisors wants to begin negotiations. Despite the valuable services these home care workers provide, they will likely suffer some form of wage and benefit cuts. Pauline realizes that those reductions in turn could have a debilitating effect on the county's senior and disabled citizens who might not receive the level of care they require.

The board of supervisors and members of the governing board want to take a hard negotiating position with the union and ask for a cut of $2.00 in the hourly wage rates of $11.50 and require workers to pay for a greater percentage of their health insurance benefits. A few supervisors think workers should cover their own health benefits given the current fiscal crisis for the county. Pauline believes this aggressive position will antagonize the president of the Local SEIU, although she thinks he must realize that the county is hurting for money and the state funding reductions are imminent. Pauline recognizes that these wage cuts might force home care workers to leave the profession to look for jobs with better wages and benefits, leaving many clients without care. As a result, these clients might end up in nursing or long-term care facilities to get the care they need, costing the county more money in the long run. The board of supervisors and Local SEIU are headed for a heated, public debate over the next few months, and Pauline will likely be in the middle of it.

Background

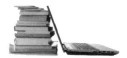

In-Home Supportive Services is a division within the California Department of Social Services of the Health and Human Services Agency. The CDSS provides services to needy children and adults through 51 offices throughout California, 58 county welfare departments, and a number of community-based organizations.[1] The IHSS program provides personal care and domestic services to persons who are elderly, disabled, or blind and who live in their own homes. These services can include household chores, food shopping, nonmedical personal care services, assistance with medications and prosthesis care, accompaniment to medical appointments, and protective supervision. The IHSS program is provided as an alternative to placement in nursing homes and long-term care facilities. As of December 2010, more than 442,000 individuals received services under the program at a monthly cost of over $400 million.[2]

IHSS is offered in every county in the State of California. Each county has an IHSS Public Authority, which is a public agency established by each respective County Board of Supervisors. The IHSS Public Authority serves low-income elderly and disabled citizens who require home care services in order to remain in their homes. The Public Authority Governing Board is advised in its recommendations by an advisory committee composed of appointed citizen members who are consumers or providers of in-home supportive services, consumer advocates, or advocates for related interested community organizations.

Next Steps

Pauline has an upcoming meeting scheduled with the executive director of the Public Authority Governing Board to discuss the proposed budget cuts. She needs to develop a social services programs funding recommendation to present to the County Board of Supervisors at its next meeting. The board of supervisors will use the recommendation as their first proposal to the SEIU to begin contract negotiations.

Discussion Questions

1. If you represented the Local SEIU, what would be your position and how would you defend it?

2. If you represented the County Board of Supervisors, what would be your position and how would you defend it?

3. Do you think the County Board of Supervisors and SEIU can reach an agreement?

4. What will be the likely public health implications of drastic budget cuts in the IHSS program?

References

[1] California Department of Social Services. (n.d.). About CDSS. Retrieved from CA.gov at http://www.dss.cahwnet.gov/cdssweb/PG190.htm

[2] California Department of Social Services. (2011, January 10). In-Home Supportive Services Management Statistics Summary Report – December. Retrieved from http://www.cdss.ca.gov/agedblinddisabled/res/pdf/2010DecMgmtStats.pdf

Case 14

CASE CONTRIBUTOR Catherine Vyskocil-Maxwell

Situation

Ms. Lukes, executive director of the Rural Prevention Network (RPN), was reviewing the agenda for the next RPN board meeting. The focus of the agenda was directly related to the sustainability plan for the RPN program, as the funding to continue the collaborative would be exhausted in the next 12 months. The agenda concluded with a summary of the plan, including action steps that would require each RPN member to provide their share of funding to continue the program. Ms. Lukes recalled that the RPN had hired her to develop and expand the RPN mission of access for the uninsured and underinsured. The program had been very successful over the past three years. She thought about the successes and barriers that had presented themselves during that time, including what had made the RPN successful in its collaboration of delivery of care to those in need.

The challenges and successes of the RPN were related to serving not only the target population but also to the partnership of the organizations with their many different nuances and leadership styles. A major challenge identified at inception was the decision not to include a hierarchy of leadership in the group, but rather to establish a level playing field in decision making. This decision presented many hurdles for Ms. Lukes, who was charged with building and strengthening relationships, designing the program, forging trust among a group of varying personalities, and driving the project forward to serve its mission of access and coordination of care for the uninsured/underinsured population. Ms. Lukes felt that these initial challenges might surface again during the next board meeting. There was an awareness of an underlying issue among board members that surfaced at the last meeting when the board member from the neighboring health system became very vocal. He was concerned about the need for a financial commitment beyond in-kind dollars for the continuation of the program. The member felt that the hosting health system (St. Peter's Health System) should fund the program, since the hosting health system was a nationally affiliated system with perceived "deep pockets." He felt there was no need for the program and that dropping all coordination of services would be acceptable to him, even though the benefits from the program were clearly documented, including reductions in non-urgent emergency room visits at member hospitals by patients in the program.

Background

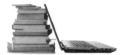

The RPN collaborative was formed in 1994 and consists of Sunrise Health Center (a federally qualified health center [FQHC]), District Health Department No. 2, Easton Area Health Center (an FQHC), Thomas City Regional Medical Center (a city-owned hospital), and St. Peter's Health System (a nonprofit hospital and the hosting member). The RPN was established for the purpose of better coordination of existing services, better accountability for quality health outcomes, and sharing resources and staff. Since 1994, the collaborative has received and successfully administered seven grants (including two grants from the Health Resources and Services Administration [HRSA], an agency of the U.S. Department of Health and Human Services) totaling $3.7 million, plus $1.7 million in local matching funds. The grants were used to address community health issues including alcohol, tobacco, drug use, teen pregnancy, and chronic disease management.

The purpose of the RPN collaborative is to improve access to and coordination of health care for the uninsured and underinsured residents in its service area by:

- Sharing relevant demographic and clinical data among all healthcare providers for this population using a shared information system;
- Engaging the medical community in a systematic and sustainable approach to care for this vulnerable population;
- Providing referrals to a primary care home and to relevant community services for this population;
- Providing individual case management services to members of the enrolled population;
- Focusing on chronic disease management; and
- Increasing access to free or discounted pharmaceuticals for the enrolled population.

The five healthcare organizations that make up the RPN entered into a formal Network Affiliation Agreement in 1994, in an effort to apply for a state community health issues grant that covered alcohol, tobacco, drug use, teen pregnancy, and chronic disease management. There was a requirement in the grant application that applicants develop a formal network of healthcare providers. The key objectives of the Network Affiliation Agreement include:

- Provide care to all individuals including the poor, underserved, uninsured, and underinsured;
- Investigate opportunities for jointly developing and integrating new and existing clinical programs and services;
- Obtain access and support in the development of administrative and clinical services as deemed necessary and appropriate to enhance service and increase efficiency by identifying and disseminating best demonstrated practices;
- Further develop and participate in managed care programs as appropriate;
- Participate in the design and implementation of an integrated delivery system development initiative;

- Explore opportunities to jointly develop programs in marketing and education; and
- Commit to develop and implement programs enhancing health status of individuals within the communities it serves.

Next Steps

Ms. Lukes felt pressure from the CEO of St. Peter's Health System to continue the program and secure funding from all the RPN collaborative members. As the hosting health system, St. Peter's Health System was her employer and the main advocate for the sustainability of the RPN. As one of the RPN group members was threatening not to fund its share, Ms. Lukes was in a tight spot. She did not know how best to maintain a cohesive attitude among the collaborative members and at the same time make sure all the members remained committed, through their continued funding, to serving those in need.

Discussion Questions

1. What should RPN do if it cannot secure funding from all members? How should it handle the likelihood that if one member does not fund, others may feel compelled to do the same?

2. What are the benefits and drawbacks for the identified healthcare organizations in developing and participating in the RPN collaborative?

3. What process should be established for the collaborative members to manage issues and conflicts that arise during its operation?

4. Given that the organization did not adopt a traditional leadership hierarchy, to whom should Ms. Lukes look for assistance in addressing the threat of one member withholding its financial support for the RPN?

Case 15

FQHC—A Cure for Ailing Community Health Centers?

CASE CONTRIBUTOR **Andrew Westrum**

Situation

The Chicago Health Alliance (CHA) is a network of four community health centers (CHCs) headquartered on Chicago's South Side: Pilsen Health Center; Hyde Park Health Center; South Chicago Health Outreach; and the Harold Washington Health Center. Each CHC provides primary care to underserved and low-income populations and specializes in the specific needs of their particular community. Hyde Park Health Center serves primarily African Americans. Pilsen Health Center primarily serves Latinos. Harold Washington Health Center serves HIV-infected individuals and provides substance abuse treatments. Southside Chicago Health Outreach serves homeless persons. Together the CHA CHCs serve more than 350,000 clients through 1,692,000 encounters annually at sites across the city. Services provided include primary medical, internal medicine, obstetrics/gynecology, pediatric, geriatric, nutrition, behavioral health, women's health, health education, and case management.

Since 2001, the CHA CHCs have worked together to integrate their healthcare services programs to more effectively and efficiently deliver quality health care. Despite their best efforts to serve each of these communities, the CHA is facing financial difficulties. Approximately 30% of the patients they serve have no health insurance and limited means to pay. The other 70% of the patients are enrolled in either Medicaid or Medicare, which also provides limited reimbursement for medical services. CHA is currently looking to the federal and state government for ways to improve their financial standing.

Background

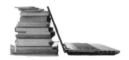

A federally qualified health center (FQHC) is a reimbursement designation, defined by the Medicare and Medicaid statutes, for all organizations receiving grants according to the Health Care Consolidation Act (Section 330 of the Public Health Service [PHS] Act). PHS 330 defines federal grant funding opportunities for organizations to provide care to underserved populations. Types of organizations that may receive PHS 330 grants include Community Health Centers, Health Care for the Homeless Programs, Migrant Health Centers, and Public Housing Primary Care Programs. FQHCs operate under the supervision of the Health Resources and Services Administration (HRSA), a key agency of the U.S. Department of Health and Human Services (HHS).

There are many benefits of being an FQHC. For FQHCs that are PHS 330 grant recipients, the biggest benefit is the grant funding. For example, new applicants may request funding up to $650,000. Other benefits include:

- Enhanced Medicaid and Medicare reimbursement;
- Access to the Vaccine for Children program managed by the Centers for Disease Control and Prevention (CDC);
- Eligibility to purchase prescription and nonprescription medications for outpatients at reduced cost through the HRSA Drug Pricing Program 340B; and
- Medical malpractice coverage through the Federal Tort Claims Act.

Next Steps

The CHA must first identify the expectations for applying for FQHC designation and match these requirements to their current healthcare services. In terms of healthcare coverage, services that must be provided directly by an FQHC or by arrangement with another provider include primary care, specialty care, dental services, mental health, substance abuse services, and transportation services necessary for adequate patient care.

HRSA also stipulates additional operating requirements, including:

- FQHCs must provide primary care services for all age groups.
- FQHCs must be open for a minimum of 32 hours per week.
- FQHCs must be open to all patients, regardless of their individual ability to pay.
- FQHCs must provide preventive health services either on site or by arrangement with another provider.
- FQHCs must use a sliding fee scale with discounts based on patient income and family size in accordance with federal poverty guidelines.

FQHCs must be either a public entity or a private nonprofit. Applications and instructions for obtaining FQHC designation may also be found on HRSA's website at http://bphc.hrsa.gov.

Discussion Questions

1. If you were the director of CHA, what would your strategy be to go about obtaining FQHC status?

2. How might you be able to determine the possible financial impact of obtaining the FQHC designation for your CHCs?

3. What other federal and state government sources might CHA look to for assistance in improving their current financial situation?

Case 16

Nonprofit Losing Funding, Not Faith

CASE CONTRIBUTOR James Christopher Middlebrook

Situation

Randall Cord is the director of Client Services for Helping Hands Home Assistance, Inc., an in-home care, nonprofit organization assisting seniors and people with physical disabilities. As a result of the current economic crisis, monetary donations to the company's SafetyNet ElderCare Program are down 20% from the year before. The SafetyNet ElderCare Program provides funding for clients to receive needed services regardless of their economic status, which allows them to continue living independently with dignity. The program is a vehicle through which organizations and individuals contribute funds for assisting this vulnerable population. Depending on the availability of funds, services are provided on a sliding-fee scale based on the client's income. If the client has no income or insurance, services are offered at no cost.

Many of the program's recipients had fallen through the cracks when searching for assistance prior to the company providing service. Randall was faced with notifying several long-term clients for whom funding was no longer available. A large number of these clients would be left with no assistance because the company has been their only source of help. Randall tried to work with other nonprofit organizations that had funding available to assist these clients or refer clients to fading state programs. Many of these clients are not able to navigate the waters of this change; therefore, Randall has been committed to advocating for clients who need help. Unfortunately, most state agencies have rigorous qualifying processes and long waiting lists, complicating the problem.

Background

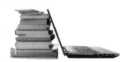

Helping Hands Home Assistance, Inc. (www.helpinghandshomeassistance.org) is a nonprofit organization serving the elderly, infirm, and those with diminished physical, intellectual, and developmental capabilities in Tennessee and Georgia. The organization provides medical and nonmedical, home-based care to assist clients with daily living so they can remain in their homes. Helping Hands Home Assistance is committed to serving those most in need, and hopes to impact the baby-boomer generation. According to the U.S. Census Bureau, by 2030 nearly 20% of the population will be 65 years and older.[1] The rapid growth of this demographic will present some challenges for nonprofit home assistance programs over the next several decades.

In the midst of Helping Hands Home Assistance being forced to cut "no-cost" services, state agencies are also reducing their programs. As state agencies face critical budget issues, many of them have cut home care services that have been shown to save money in the long run, because fewer people are being sent to more costly nursing homes.[2] Presently, nursing homes are big businesses with more political power and are in direct competition with smaller nonprofit organizations.

Given funding cutbacks and the economic downturn, the neediest in society are being left to fend for themselves as overwhelmed nonprofit staff struggle to meet the needs of their clients. Helping Hands Home Assistance and its staff have pledged not to give up, and have looked to the public health community to help rescue those in need.

Next Steps

Due to current economic pressures, Randall met with his employees, challenging them to generate fund-raising activities in order to continue service provision for indigent clients. The staff conceived events such as a communitywide benefit dinner, at which resident companies and citizens purchased tickets to a gala showcasing care recipients who gave heartfelt testimonials of how this program benefited them.

This event and other fundraisers continue to be the lifeblood for providing help to clients who are unable to acquire help from other programs. Randall and his team work tirelessly to keep clients funded for services. Even so, the nonprofit organization was not able to serve all of its long-term clientele, forcing some clients into state-administered programs.

Discussion Questions

1. What role should government public health agencies have to help protect quality of life for seniors and people with physical disabilities who are in need of home care services?

2. What methods should public health officials use to optimize welfare provisions, including increasing funding and scrutinizing inappropriate and illegal use, even if such methods add to the overall costs of administering such programs?

3. How does governmental oversight facilitate or inhibit administration of home care assistance programs?

4. What can Randall do to help raise funding for his organization and in turn help his clients?

5. How does moving clientele from private, nonprofit organizations to more expensive state-administered programs affect the long-term viability of public health agencies?

References

[1] U.S. Census Bureau. (n.d.). U.S. population projections [Table 3: Ranking of states by projected percent of population age 65 and over: 2000, 2010, and 2030]. Retrieved from http://www.census .gov/population/www/projections/projectionsagesex.html

[2] Leland, J. (2010, July 20). Cuts in home care put elderly and disabled at risk. *The New York Times*. Retrieved from http://www.nytimes.com/2010/07/21/us/21aging.html

Case 17

Beyond a Patient Complaint

CASE CONTRIBUTOR **Beth Ann Taylor**

Situation

Dr. Camille Smith is reviewing a patient complaint file in preparation for a meeting with the key physicians and her pharmacy chief. Dr. Smith works for a federally funded community health center and as director must lead a discussion session with her team that will generate a recommended approach to address this concern. The team will need to not only look at this patient, but will also need to establish an approach for addressing all similar concerns in the population they serve. As Dr. Smith ponders the situation, she is concerned about the financial implications of the decision, knowing the potential costs.

Background

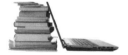

Mr. Alfred Jones, a 66-year-old retiree who has been receiving care at this facility for the last decade, submitted a complaint about his physician, which resulted in this review. Mr. Jones has a history of high blood pressure, diabetes, and mild arthritis and agrees that his physician has helped him manage these issues very well. However, Mr. Jones has recently accused the physician, Dr. Franklin Mitchell, of withholding proper treatment from him by not prescribing a medication that he is certain would alleviate one of his health problems and assist him in becoming fully functional. He now believes he is being denied a medication that will improve his quality of life. He has become so angry that he sent not only a letter of complaint to Dr. Smith but to his local paper, other patients of the clinic, and congressional representatives.

Dr. Mitchell has been caring for Mr. Jones since he began coming to the clinic and believed they had a positive working relationship until recently. Since his retirement, Mr. Jones spends most of his time watching TV and browsing the Internet focusing on sites related to his health issues and has become increasingly insistent on receiving certain medications he has "researched." Dr. Mitchell believes his latest request for an expensive non-formulary medication, which will not improve or mitigate any of his health issues, is not a good expenditure of funds and is refusing to write a prescription demanded by Mr. Jones.

Next Steps

As he prepares for the meeting with Dr. Smith, Dr. Mitchell wants to discuss how to maximize the health and happiness of his patients while being a good steward of the facility's financial resources.

Discussion Questions

1. How do the interests of Dr. Smith, Mr. Jones, and Dr. Mitchell differ? How are they similar?

2. What are the implications of their decision for the population served?

3. What are the implications of their decision for the individual patient?

4. How might the physicians be affected by their decision?

5. Describe the leadership approach Dr. Smith should take with her team.

Group Exercise

Select three students to role-play Dr. Smith, Mr. Jones, and Dr. Mitchell. Dr. Smith is to meet with both the physician and the patient separately. In the role play she is to listen and respond to each. Student observers are to look for body language, nonverbal and verbal communication, and provide feedback as to her effectiveness as a leader/manager.

Case 18   Building Latrines—Half the Solution to Global Sanitation

CASE CONTRIBUTOR James K. Arinaitwe

Situation

Global Health Initiative (GHI) is a network of volunteers, professionals, and students who partner with grassroots organizations and communities to improve the health and well-being of people living in poverty. GHI has chapters across 40 U.S. states and over 44 grassroots partner organizations in developing countries. The Florida State University chapter of GHI advocates for better community and individual health for the people of Orissa, India.

For generations, the people of Orissa have used bushes and ponds to relieve themselves of their excrement. As populations grew and environmental circumstances such as flooding occurred, this has caused huge outbreaks of diseases such as cholera, dysentery, diarrhea, and many parasitic infections. These diseases are all due to drinking fecal-contaminated water. As a solution to the sanitation and health problems of Orissa, the Tallahassee-based chapter of GHI is charged with raising enough funds to construct at least 1000 latrines by 2015; that is 200 latrines per year, beginning in 2011.

Solomon is the GHI's global health director in Florida. His responsibility is to galvanize colleagues and find fundraising strategies that will raise a total of $800,000 to cover the costs of $800 per latrine for the community of Orissa.

Background

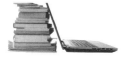

For generations, the people of Orissa have lived without sanitation and have used nearby fields, ponds, and roadsides as their toilets. But the sanitation movement is sweeping across not only Orissa, but also in the West Bengal area. The habits of a lifetime are changing, the hopes of sanitation are increasing, and the cases of diarrhea and other fecal-contamination diseases are falling. The success of GHI's public health campaign to include latrines in every household by 2015 would rapidly reduce the cases of diarrhea, dysentery, and cholera.

Building latrines in Orissa will not solve all their problems, as those in rural India are the poorest of the poor. Education campaigns in both private and public schools are necessary to sensitize these communities about the needs of proper sanitation and better hygiene practices. These efforts need to be employed by donors, local governments, nongovernmental organizations, and communities in order for the sanitation initiative to take root in rural India. The challenges faced by GHI's latrine campaign are enormous; however, there are two that are eminent: (1) rejection of the new latrines by the elderly who are stuck in their old ways of life and who still consider sanitation a "dirty word" and (2) latrines filling up (for extended families) sooner and having to move them to another location, which would take up another piece of land necessary for agriculture.

Next Steps

Solomon is optimistic that by scheduling bimonthly meetings, one with the people of Orissa and the other with his team in Florida, his team and the people of Orissa will meet both their financial and sanitation goals for those in rural India.

Discussion Questions

1. Outline fundraising strategies that Solomon and his team could employ to meet their financial goals.

2. In rural India, as in other developing regions, how can latrines be implemented in spite of rejections by older generations who see them as intrusive to their old ways of life?

3. Due to population growth, latrines have been found to fill up quickly and overflow. This requires another hole to be dug, using even more land, which is a scarce resource. How can this problem be solved (think of sustainable, eco-friendly solutions)?

4. GHI relies on the strength of donors and fundraisers to meet the global health challenges in rural communities of developing countries. In what ways could GHI work to wean these communities off dependency on foreign support in order to initiate their own solutions to their public health needs?

5. What are some other solutions to global sanitation that public health organizations and volunteers can address?

Case 19

Numbers and Degrees—Challenges for the Nursing Workforce

CASE CONTRIBUTOR **Kay Wagner**

Situation

In 2008, the Robert Wood Johnson Foundation (RWJF) partnered with the Institute of Medicine (IOM) to produce a report that would make recommendations for the profession of nursing. The 2010 report, *The Future of Nursing: Leading Change, Advancing Health,* made eight recommendations, the fourth of which was to increase the proportion of nurses with a baccalaureate degree from 50% to 80% by 2020.[1] Since 1970, the IOM has historically provided unbiased and authoritative advice to improve the overall health of the United States and often becomes the impetus for change in the nation's health care as was the case with the 1999 report *To Err Is Human.*

A dichotomy exists with the above-mentioned recommendation and the fact that there is a current nursing faculty shortage in academia coupled with a projected nursing shortage in the near future. According to the U.S. Department of Labor, registered nurses (RNs) are projected to add the most jobs of any other occupation, with 582,000 more RNs needed by 2018 (a 22.2% increase from 2008).[2] In the hospital setting alone, nurses account for the largest component of staff. Federal projections show a demand for RNs in the hospital setting rising by 36% by 2020.[3]

Nancy, the Workforce Development Coordinator for MidMichigan Health, is responsible for the oversight of all nursing workforce initiatives across the system. She is well aware of the significance of the IOM report and the challenges that lie ahead for the profession. Current economic conditions are making it difficult for eligible RNs to retire due to retirement investment losses and an increase in the cost of living, which equates to an older workforce whose degrees are primarily from associate or diploma programs. This adds to the issue of having too few nurses with bachelor of science in nursing (BSN) degrees in the workforce. Research shows that a higher proportion of BSN-prepared or higher educated RNs has been shown to decrease surgical patient mortality.[4] In addition to a sluggish economy, healthcare reform is putting a financial strain on many healthcare organizations as a result of the Patient Protection and Affordable Care Act and the National Strategy for Quality Improvement in Health Care, which enforces more stringent reimbursements based on quality of care versus quantity. The workforce development budget for MidMichigan Health, which includes monies for tuition reimbursement, nurse externship, nurse residency, and nurse preceptor programs, has remained flat, been reduced, or been placed on hold. All of these variables contribute to the main issues facing the nursing workforce: too few numbers and too few nurses with BSN degrees.

Background

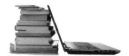

MidMichigan Health is a nonprofit health system, headquartered in Midland, Michigan. It covers a 12-county region with medical centers in Midland, Alma, Clare, and Gladwin, as well as urgent care centers, home care, long-term care, physician groups, medical offices, and other specialty health services. MidMichigan Health has more than 6,000 employees, physicians, and volunteers. Approximately 800 of these employees are RNs who are providing direct care at the bedside with varying degrees (associate two year, diploma three year, and baccalaureate four year). The academic institutions that serve as the RN pipeline for the health system at a regional level consist of three universities with baccalaureate degree programs and four community colleges with associate degree programs. Nancy serves on all of the academic nursing advisory boards. These boards consist of members from the healthcare organizations who are charged with providing feedback to the academic institutions with regards to curriculum development and programs that meet the needs of the organizations. As a participant in the board meetings, Nancy has evidenced an increasing focus on the nursing workforce issues specific to the IOM report recommendations. From a recruitment perspective, in addition to MidMichigan Health, graduates can select from four other acute care hospitals within a 30-mile radius of any one of the MidMichigan Health affiliates. This competition limits the overall pool of BSN-prepared graduates for hire by MidMichigan Health.

MidMichigan Health has participated in various initiatives to advance the education of its nursing population. It was recently recognized as the recipient of the 2011 Building Michigan's Healthcare Workforce Michigan Health Council Award in the category of Regional Collaboration (www.mhc.org/bmhw_award.php) for such initiatives, which included partnering with universities for onsite RN to BSN completion programs, a licensed practical nurse (LPN) to RN completion program in collaboration with a partnering community college with 20 seats reserved for MidMichigan Health LPNs, and a grant recipient and participant in the RWJF Partners Investing in Nursing's (PIN) Future program. The PIN program was a collaborative project that produced 13 additional master of science in nursing (MSN) prepared RNs for the region.

Next Steps

Nancy has been asked by the vice president of Human Resources to investigate the IOM report in more detail and work with the necessary stakeholders to develop a strategic plan to advance the education of the current RN workforce for the health system. The plan will be shared with the administrative team, board members, and academic partners. She is to perform a strengths, weaknesses, opportunities, and threats (SWOT) analysis of the current RN workforce, including information at an organizational, system, and regional level to help develop her plan and make recommendations. Nancy has identified the following key variables to consider:

- Currently, there is no wage differentiation for RNs based on degrees within the system.

- A magnet healthcare organization (i.e., it has an American Nurses Credentialing Center designation, which recognizes healthcare organizations for quality patient care, nursing excellence, and innovations) in Michigan has recently taken a bold step in transitioning to an all-BSN hiring practice.
- As recently as five years ago, MidMichigan Health faced a shortage of more than 50 RNs throughout the system. The majority of those positions were filled with associate degree RNs due to the limited number of BSN graduates in the region.

Discussion Questions

1. Identify the key stakeholders that Nancy must consider in preparing her strategic plan.

2. What are the key considerations for Nancy in recommending an all-BSN RN workforce for the future of MidMichigan Health?

3. If MidMichigan Health pursues an all-BSN RN workforce, what cultural challenges might the system encounter? How might the system proactively manage such challenges?

4. What obligation, if any, does MidMichigan Health have to its existing nurses who do not have BSN degrees and yet could have many more years of service left with the system?

5. Identify a desirable outcome of Nancy's strategic plan and describe a benchmark that can measure the success of meeting the selected outcome.

References

[1] Institute of Medicine. (2010). *The future of nursing: Leading change, advancing health*. Retrieved from http://www.iom.edu/~/media/Files/Report%20Files/2010/The-Future-of-Nursing/Future%20 of%20Nursing%202010%20Recommendations.pdf

[2] United States Department of Labor Bureau of Labor Statistics. (2009). Economic news release. Employment projections: 2008–2018 summary. Retrieved from http://www.bls.gov/news.release/ ecopro.nr0.htm

[3] American Association of Colleges of Nursing. (2011). Nursing fact sheet. Retrieved from http:// www.aacn.nche.edu/media-relations/fact-sheets/nursing-fact-sheet

[4] Aiken, L. H., Clarke, S. P., Cheung, R. B., Sloane, D. M., & Silber, J. H. (2003). Educational levels of hospital nurses and surgical patient mortality. *JAMA, 290*(12), 1617–1623.

Case 20 | Orienting a Contract Physical Therapist

CASE CONTRIBUTOR Emily van de Water

Situation

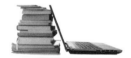

Peter is the rehabilitation director at Palm Springs Medical Center in Palm Springs, California. Among other duties, he is responsible for hiring new physical, occupational, and speech therapists to treat patients in the outpatient clinic and hospital. The physical therapy patient load is high, and Peter knows he has to hire another physical therapist in the clinic. He decides to hire a contract physical therapist to meet the demand in the near term.

Background

Contract therapists, or traveling therapists as they are known, generally work 13-week contract jobs and move around within a state and/or country for different positions where there is extra or temporary demand for additional therapists (e.g., filling in for therapists on maternity or medical leaves). They work for an agency that specializes in finding these contract positions and recruiting nurses, physical therapists, occupational therapists, and speech therapists to fill them. Positions for traveling therapists are available in most clinical settings, including hospitals, outpatient clinics, and schools. Contract therapists are paid stipends by their employers to cover housing and meal expenses while on assignment. Recruiters who place contract workers are also paid for their services. Therefore, these types of workers cost more to hire than permanent workers. Prior to signing a contract, all parties negotiate the payment package.

Contract therapists seek out such assignments to try out new locations and types of facilities. A requirement of the job, however, is that they have to be flexible in adjusting to a new workplace while also learning the culture and practices of a new clinical setting. The adjustment process can be frustrating at times, however, as Peter experienced with his last contract therapist. The State of California requires physical therapists to have a background check and be fingerprinted prior to issuing a license. The last therapist was fingerprinted twice on paper and once via Live Scan (a digital fingerprint). However, due to technical issues, her fingerprints were rejected under both methods. It took the Department of Justice in California 45 days to complete a "name verification" before it could issue a license. Luckily, the State of California has a Physical Therapist License Applicant status, which allowed the therapist to practice until the licensed was issued, but she had to have another full-time therapist co-sign her treatment notes.

Next Steps

Peter contacts Travel Medical, a company that has placed traveling therapists at his hospital in the past, to inform them about the position and asks if they have any travelers who are looking for a job in the Palm Springs area. He interviews three candidates over the phone and offers the job to Jane, as she has the most experience in outpatient physical therapy settings. Jane will be relocating from Jacksonville, FL, and will begin working at the hospital in three weeks.

Discussion Questions

1. How should Peter help prepare Jane for working at the clinic before she arrives?

2. Knowing Jane's situation, what would you include in Jane's orientation to the clinic?

3. Typically, therapists are treating 10–12 patients per day. Since Jane will have to learn the administrative processes of the job as well, what should her patient load look like for the first week?

4. Given present workforce shortages in the healthcare industry, how should healthcare administrators prepare and manage their work environment for the regular use of contract employees?

5. What cultural challenges must an administrator consider as contract employees become more common in the healthcare workforce?

Case 21 — Revamping Ineffective Performance Reviews

CASE CONTRIBUTOR **Kathleen M. Reville**

Situation

Richard and Kate were finishing their lunch and discussing their performance reviews, which had taken place that morning. Richard, the director of Clinical Services at West Bridgewater Health Center, was relaying the details of his performance improvement plan and his excitement with his supervisor's allocation of some professional development time. Kate, manager of Outpatient Services, sat dumbfounded. Her performance review consisted of a series of average scores, combined with the threat of better performance "or else." While Richard and Kate were talking, it became apparent that they were both lacking skills in the same area, time management, and yet their supervisors' approaches had been dramatically different with each. Richard felt like he had the support of his supervisor to make necessary improvements through professional development opportunities, while Kate felt demoralized and humiliated. How could two similar performance reviews have had two such different outcomes?

Background

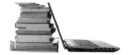

Annual performance reviews create anxiety and are rarely used effectively. They are often treated as a necessary evil, when they could be used as an important tool to further develop staff competencies. In addition, many managers avoid having difficult conversations with staff because this creates an uncomfortable situation or they are afraid of legal ramifications. Axline, a scholar in business ethics, states, "The overall objective of high-ethics performance review should be to provide an honest assessment of performance and to mutually develop a plan to improve the individual's effectiveness. That requires telling people where they stand and being straight with them."[1] When performance reviews are not being conducted effectively, the entire organization suffers and staff is left without important and honest feedback about their performance.

Next Steps

The organization should create a culture that values and utilizes performance reviews. Often, the review tools become stale and outdated. The first step for the human resources director is to review these tools with managers and staff to determine whether the tool itself could be improved to lead to more honest feedback. Once this review is completed, managers should be trained on the new tool as well as coached on effective performance review techniques. The organization should provide follow-up training as well as track the effectiveness of the new measures to ensure impact.

Discussion Questions

1. What should Kate do to follow up on her performance review? Would it be helpful for her to have a conversation with her supervisor?

2. If you were Kate's supervisor and the issue was time management, how would you present a more encouraging performance evaluation?

3. As human resources director, describe a training program that you would provide to Kate's supervisor to create a more participatory review process.

Reference

[1] Axline, L. L. (1996, Winter). The ethics of performance appraisal. *Advanced Management Journal, 61*(1), 44–45. Retrieved from Academic OneFile.

Case 22

CASE CONTRIBUTOR **James A. Johnson**

Situation

Amherst Psychiatric Institute's nursing staff is composed of nurses and mental health counselors who provide 24-hour direct inpatient care.[1] All nurses at Amherst have a state license and one of three educational accomplishments: a two-year hospital-based nursing diploma, a two-year associate degree in nursing, or a four-year bachelor's degree in nursing. All mental health counselors are required to have a four-year bachelor's degree, preferably in the social science field, and some hold master's degrees in psychology.

The job responsibilities of the nurses and counselors are quite similar. In addition to their primary role of establishing a therapeutic relationship with patients, mental health counselors, like nurses, are required to take vital signs, give bed baths, assist with patients' activities of daily living (ADLs), and administer catheters as needed. Because the psychiatric patient usually requires less invasive therapy and supportive care than do medical/ surgical patients, few distinctions are noticed in the routine function of the staff. Working relationships between the nurses and counselors appear harmonious most of the time. Minor conflicts over job duties are quickly and quietly resolved by the unit nurse manager.

For the past year, the attrition rate among the counselors has been increasing steadily, but neither the unit nurse manager nor the director of nursing for the department has questioned the staff about the possible reasons for the turnover. Vacancies are usually filled immediately to adjust the patient-to-staff ratio. The unit nurse manager informs the mental health counselor applicants that (a) the position does not offer an opportunity for career advancement within the department; (b) a working unity exists between the nurses and counselors to coordinate and deliver quality care; and (c) staff members are encouraged to resolve their own conflicts before approaching management.

Next Steps

Unbeknownst to staff members and the nursing administration, the mental health counselors have formed a separate action group outside the work environment to discuss their dissatisfaction concerning their roles and responsibilities and the conflicts that exist with the staff nurses. They share a common feeling of perceived lack of value by the nurses and administration. The counselors have agreed to present the problems affecting their morale and job performance to the nursing staff and administration and have chosen a spokesperson to voice their concerns at a meeting of counselors, nurses, and administration. The presentation follows.

> We, the mental health counselors, are confused about our role within the nursing department. We perceive that we are made to feel subordinate to nurses in patient

care areas such as counseling, even though many of us have a wealth of knowledge and experience in this area of patient care. We feel our efforts are undervalued and often go unrecognized by the nursing administration.

We do not want to take anything away from the nurses; rather, we would like to share equally in those areas of patient care in which we are qualified. It appears as if the administration continually seeks ways to expand and empower the role of nurses while excluding counselors from consideration for duties that may require more authority. Indeed our responsibilities at times have been further diminished. For many years, mental health counselors were responsible for processing patient admission and discharge procedures except for gathering intake physical information and examinations. Suddenly, we were given notice not to administer these responsibilities because of The Joint Commission's requirement that an RN must perform and document these duties. Yet our requests for documentation to support this change went unanswered, and now, six months later, we have been allowed to resume these duties without an explanation.

We are led to believe that nurses, like mental health counselors, share similar duties for the caring of patients. We also recognize that some techniques and interventions are specific for nurses; however, when daily assignments are made for patient care, mental health counselors inevitably are assigned to bedridden patients who require primary nursing care. We expected a sharing of duties. During our staff retreat, an announcement was made to staff nurses and mental health counselors about a possible pay increase of $1.00 an hour to occur soon. Later, we learned that only nurses were granted this raise. Again, no consideration was given to counselors as valued members of the nursing department.

Memos addressed to "All Nursing Staff" are passed individually to nurses. Counselors are left to learn of department policy changes through staff nurses.

Participation in team meetings is another area in which we feel we are unfairly excluded. Although these meetings are said to be open to counselors, in reality we are left to staff the unit while nurses attend the meetings. How are we to be team members when we share unequally in the team process?

As one mental health counselor expressed, "I don't think the nurses respect and trust our decision making. In a way their actions indicate we are not qualified. In fact, on matters of assessing a patient's mental health, I am equally if not more qualified to address these concerns than are the staff nurses." If we are to be members of the nursing staff and work together to provide quality patient care, we need to be heard and made a part of the decision-making process. Along these same lines, when we report on a patient's behavioral condition, we are often ignored. Possibly a communication conflict exists. The element of trust is a vital component of the communication process.

We want and need your input to bridge the gap we perceive exists. We want to listen and hear from you too. Our goal is not to create a rift between us, but to merge and complement each other's skills and abilities to structure a proud and caring nursing staff.

Discussion Questions

1. If you were the nursing director, how would you respond to the counselors' plea and the covert way in which it was formed?

2. How do you think the nurses, administration, and other managers will respond to these allegations of inequality?

3. What actions will you take to meet the requests of your counselors?

4. What implications will this request have on the (a) relationship between nurses and counselors, (b) relationship between staff and management, (c) existing department policies, (d) job descriptions of both nurses and counselors, and (e) hiring practices?

Reference

[1] Kilpatrick, A. O., & Johnson, J. A. (1999). *Human resources and organizational behavior: Cases in health services management*. Chicago: Health Administration Press.

Case 23

A Case of Reverse Discrimination?

CASE CONTRIBUTOR Scott D. Musch

Situation

NPMC Care Clinic (NPMC) provides community-based primary care to adults requiring specialized health care and social services in North Philadelphia. The clinic operates under the guidance of St. Joseph's Hospital in North Philadelphia and offers medical services, support services, and medical case management. Brad, a recent graduate from the Boston University School of Social Work, joined NPMC six months ago as a case manager in the HIV/AIDS Services Program. Brad earned his master's in Social Work and wants to become certified as a licensed clinical social worker (LCSW). He enjoys performing HIV/AIDs social work as he finds it extremely rewarding. Most individuals with AIDS are poor and must rely on the limited benefits of public health insurance and usually cannot afford to purchase additional services when they are needed. Case managers help people living with HIV/AIDS get primary medical care and medications, adhere to treatment plans, and access supportive services such as housing, transportation, food, and mental health counseling. As an LCSW, Brad would develop comprehensive, individualized care plans for clients and work closely with other team members in the clinic to ensure his client's medical, mental health, and social services are being addressed. As part of the licensure requirements in Pennsylvania, Brad needs to complete three years or 3000 hours of supervised work experience in a clinical setting. Brad was excited to join NPMC as it had an active patient case load and his supervisor seemed eager to help him work toward his licensure requirements.

In the HIV Services Program at NPMC, Brad works closely with two other case managers, Tim and Michael, who have been with the clinic for approximately two years. His working relationship with his colleagues was at first very amicable. He seemed to be accepted by them and at times they joked with him for being the "straight advocate" or "token" in their group. Tim and Michael are gay, as is the supervisor of the program, while Brad is heterosexual. Tim and Michael are open about their sexual orientation, and while Brad doesn't feel uncomfortable, at times he doesn't understand their humor. Tim and Michael would often share their dating adventures of their previous night's encounters in the office and Brad would look forward to hearing their humorous stories. Brad enjoyed conversing with his colleagues. He also had a good initial relationship with his boss. His supervisor was well respected in the department and he offered Brad much encouragement. Gradually, Brad noticed that his supervisor seemed more inclined toward Tim and Michael, but he didn't make much out of it as he figured it was probably due to their being able to relate better given their shared culture.

After five months, however, the general atmosphere at work changed. Brad felt increasingly like an outsider. While the case load at NPMC was fairly distributed, Brad's cases seemed to get less attention from his supervisor than Tim's and Michael's cases. The majority of Brad's patients were heterosexual and he sensed reluctance on the part of his supervisor to assign him more cases involving gay patients. From Brad's perspective, Tim and Michael seemed busier and their cases tended to receive more exposure throughout the clinic. Brad tried to defuse his impression of the situation by approaching his supervisor to volunteer to handle a greater "variety" of cases. However, while his supervisor acknowledged his interest, he told Brad that Tim and Michael had a more appropriate background to handle these types of cases. Brad tried to dismiss his concerns over the apparent favoritism in the office and focused on doing his work. Adding to his suspicions of favoritism, Brad often found Tim and Michael in his supervisor's office in what appeared to be formal meetings. On occasion, Brad tried to join these meetings by hanging outside his supervisor's office door to give the impression of wanting to be involved. His supervisor would call him in and generally didn't seem to mind; however, he never directly addressed Brad's lack of invitation. Gradually, Brad stopped making the extra effort to be involved and just concentrated on his case load at his desk.

Brad's relations with his colleagues Tim and Michael grew increasingly strained. What was once a collegial atmosphere in the office was now tense. Tim and Michael no longer included him in their "water-cooler" talk and even if he tried to join in, they seemed to tense up and shortly end their lively discussions. On several occasions, Brad thought he heard Tim and Michael making off-handed comments about him, referring to him as the "breeder" in the office. In addition, they seemed particularly extra-sensitive to any comments Brad might make that appeared critical of their behavior, including comments on risky sexual behaviors that he may have relayed from a patient case. Brad felt increasingly isolated in the office. He tried to dismiss his concerns as just "being in his head" as he really needed the hours at the clinic to meet his goal of obtaining his license.

Background

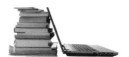

Federal laws prohibit discrimination based on race, color, sex, religion, national origin, age, and disability for private employers. Sex discrimination claims by workers are most often filed under Title VII of the Civil Rights Act of 1964 (Pub. L. 88-352).[1] Sexual discrimination prohibited under Title VII includes discrimination based on pregnancy, sex stereotyping, and sexual harassment. Title VII does not prohibit discrimination based on sexual orientation though some state discrimination laws do. Almost half of the U.S. states, including the District of Columbia, have active laws that prohibit sexual orientation discrimination in both private and public workplaces. A few states prohibit sexual orientation discrimination in only public workplaces, such as for state employees, as is the case with Pennsylvania (as of 2010). Sexual orientation discrimination involves a situation when someone is treated differently solely because of his or her sexual orientation: gay (homosexual), lesbian, bisexual, or straight (heterosexual). This type of discrimination may also occur on the basis of a perception of someone's orientation, whether that perception is correct or not. The Employment Non-Discrimination Act (ENDA) proposed federal legislation that would add sexual orientation as a protected class against discrimination.[2]

While ENDA has been proposed in the U.S. Congress numerous times, it has failed to pass. Sexual harassment is a form of sex discrimination that is prohibited by federal law and the law of most states, regardless of whether the state also has a law making discrimination on the basis of sexual orientation illegal. The victim as well as the harasser may be a woman or a man, and the victim does not have to be of the opposite sex to be able to bring a legal claim for sexual harassment.

Next Steps

Brad once looked forward to getting up in the morning and going to work. He really had a passion for helping his clients. However, increasingly he had to drag himself out of bed. He felt isolated and dreaded having to face his colleagues in the office. He knew he had to address the situation as he didn't want it to start to affect his love for social work. He considered meeting with NPMC's human resources director. What would he say? There wasn't any direct evidence on which to build a case for discrimination. Who would believe that a heterosexual male among gay workers could be the object of discrimination? Brad believed the human resources director was also gay, so he wasn't confident he would get a fair hearing. His perceptions would probably just be dismissed as paranoid. In addition, if his supervisor found out about his meeting with human resources, the situation would only become worse. Brad thought that it might be time to look seriously for another job.

Discussion Questions

1. What should Brad do?

2. If you were the HR director, what issues would you address?

3. Is Brad a victim of reverse discrimination?

4. How might Brad's supervisor make for a more inclusive work environment?

References

[1] U.S. Equal Employment Opportunity Commission. (n.d.). Title VII of the Civil Rights Act of 1964. Retrieved from http://www.eeoc.gov/laws/statutes/titlevii.cfm

[2] Employment Non-Discrimination Act of 2009, H.R. 3017, 111th Congress. (2009–2010). Retrieved from http://www.govtrack.us/congress/bill.xpd?bill=h111-3017

Case 24

Sexual Harassment at St. Catherine

CASE CONTRIBUTOR **James A. Johnson**

Situation

Fatima was hired as a registered nurse in the maternity department of St. Catherine Hospital on July 1, immediately after her graduation from nursing school.[1] Her husband, Ali, had been working as a lab technician at St. Catherine for more than five years. Fatima was happy with her job and enjoyed socializing with her coworkers. Her only complaint was that she was assigned to the night shift while her husband worked the day shift.

After Fatima had been working at St. Catherine for three months, Ali asked his boss to speak to the hospital director about the possibility of getting Fatima reassigned to the day shift. He did, and two days later Fatima's shift was changed. When Omar, the nursing supervisor, heard about the change in Fatima's work schedule, he was angry that he had not been included in the decision-making process. He also began to pay attention to Fatima for the first time since she began working at St. Catherine. Omar began making unusually frequent visits to the maternity department, especially the area where Fatima worked. The head nurse in the maternity department, Anne, noticed the frequent visits but didn't speculate about the reason for them.

On October 20, Omar called Fatima into his office. They had the following conversation:

Omar: I asked you to come here so I could find out more about you before assigning you more responsibility.

Fatima: More responsibility? What do you mean?

Omar: Well, I was thinking of promoting you to head nurse of the maternity department.

Fatima: Head nurse? Anne is more qualified for that position than I am; she has far more experience. Besides, I need to work here for at least one year before I'm eligible for a promotion.

Omar: I know the rules. But, you see, I have a lot of influence at the hospital. I can persuade the director very easily. Besides, Anne has a record of being hostile toward hospital administration.

Fatima: Thank you for the offer, but I don't think I'm qualified for the position. I need to get back to my work now, if we're finished here.

Omar: OK, but give my offer some more thought. This is a great opportunity for you, and I don't want you to miss it because I care for you. Oh, one more thing, could you please keep this conversation confidential?

After this conversation, Omar's visits to the maternity department became even more frequent. On November 15, Omar came to the department at 6 p.m., after most of the nurses had gone home. Fatima was still there, getting ready to leave.

Omar: I'm glad you're alone. I just want to ask if you have some free time next week. I'd like us to spend some time together . . . .

Fatima: Stop it! You are my supervisor, and you are supposed to set an example of honesty and respect. Besides, we're both married. Please excuse me; my husband is waiting for me.

Fatima left the hospital feeling upset and embarrassed. Because of her religious and social beliefs, however, she chose not to tell anybody about what happened, even her husband. The following day, still upset, she called in sick. Omar, angry, immediately reported her absence to the director.

Next Steps

One week later, Fatima was transferred to the intensive care unit and a written warning was placed in her permanent record. Fatima, with only a few months of nursing experience, was not prepared for the complexity of the work in her new position. The head nurse of the intensive care unit, Renee, was instructed by Omar to notify him in writing of every instance in which Fatima was not able to perform her new duties. Omar provided the discipline committee with copies of these documents and used them to convince the members of the committee that Fatima had failed to carry out her assignments properly. As a result, Fatima was transferred to a small rural hospital located 95 miles from St. Catherine.

In July, at the end of her first year of employment, Fatima received a copy of her performance evaluation. It stated, "After a one-year probationary period, Fatima's performance did not meet the necessary requirements; therefore, we are recommending the prolongation of her probationary period for an additional year." The performance evaluation was signed by the director of St. Catherine, Omar, and Renee. Fatima refused to sign and decided to file official sexual harassment charges against Omar.

Discussion Questions

1. How could this situation have been handled differently?

2. Is Omar the only person at fault in this case? Do the head nurses and hospital director share in any of the responsibility?

3. If you were assigned responsibility to research this case, what kinds of questions would you ask the parties involved?

Reference

[1] Kilpatrick, A. O., & Johnson, J. A. (1999). *Human resources and organizational behavior: Cases in health services management.* Chicago: Health Administration Press.

Case 25

CASE CONTRIBUTOR Scott D. Musch

Situation

"Stephen just quit," Betty interjected as Katherine walked by the desk. "Apparently, he felt frustrated in his job. He found an opportunity with more responsibility at Riverside Health Clinic." Katherine, the human resources director for the State Department of Health and Environmental Control (DHEC), paused and absorbed the news. "Stephen is the third employee to leave the Program Department in the last 12 months," Katherine replied. "Why can't Bill hold on to his younger employees?" She thought there must be more behind the departures than simply better opportunities.

Stephen had worked in the central office of the Public Health Programs department under the supervision of Bill, a 30-year veteran with the DHEC. The department oversaw and coordinated program initiatives for three branches: Health Services, Health Regulations, and Environmental Control. Bill supervised approximately 25 employees in various capacities, including three managers with responsibility for programs in each of the three branches. Bill had worked his way up through the organization, starting his career at a local health department within the state and eventually earning his current position. Bill was a seasoned professional within the DHEC with a wide breadth of experience and he had a strict, almost authoritarian, management style. The three other managers were also long-term employees with an average tenure of 20 years. On the other hand, Stephen was a recent undergraduate recruit from a well-respected school of public health. The other two employees who resigned were also relatively young employees, having worked in the department for less than two years.

Katherine had spoken with Bill after the other two employees departed. Katherine felt that Bill needed to reevaluate his management style and recognize how his workforce was changing, particularly with the millennial generation, adults who were born after 1982 and are just now starting to enter the workforce in greater numbers (see Figure 25–1). However, Bill was resistant. He echoed a comment that she often heard from other managers in the office: "Why do we need to change our culture for these new employees?"

Figure 25–1 Generations

Generation	Veterans	Baby Boomers	Generation X	Millennial
Years born	1925–1942	1943–1964	1965–1981*	1982*–2002
Ages in 2011	69–86	47–68	30–46	9–29

© Cengage Learning 2013

*Sources differ on end and beginning dates

Background

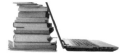

In its report, *Confronting the Public Health Workforce Crisis*, the Association of Schools of Public Health (ASPH) estimated that 250,000 additional public health workers will be needed by 2020, largely attributed to the current workforce slowly diminishing as approximately 23% will be eligible to retire by 2012.[1] For some state health agencies, this percentage is more drastic, reaching over 50% as reported in the Association of State and Territorial Health Officials' *2007 State Public Health Workforce Shortage Report*.[2] To replenish the workforce and avert a crisis, the ASPH estimates that schools of public health will need to train three times the current number of graduates over the next 11 years.[1] While there are many implications from these statistics, one is clear: the public health workforce will gradually be younger and employees from the millennial generation will become a larger part of the workforce.

The multigenerational workforce in public health, as with all industries, presents numerous challenges. While casting stereotypes within any demographic group can lead to simplistic conclusions, each generation has a slightly different paradigm for the role of work in life and the standards for that work. Employers who understand how each generation's values, ethics, and expectations affect the workplace may be able to better optimize employee productivity, retention, and success. Incorporating this understanding into management practices may reduce generational conflict and miscommunication. Much has been written on the subject of the millennial generation, including recommended techniques for recruiting, managing, motivating, and retaining these employees. Among the research, some general characteristics are apparent. Desirable attributes in a job for millennials include a preference for an inclusive work environment, team collaboration, challenges and opportunities to learn new skills, flexibility, and life–work balance. Employers tend to go wrong with millennials when they do not provide clear growth opportunities, discount their ideas for lack of experience, and feel threatened by their technical knowledge.

Next Steps

Sitting in her office, Katherine reflects on the loss of another employee in Bill's department. As a human resources professional, Katherine has come across many articles and presentations on the topic of the millennial workforce and related challenges of a multigenerational workforce. With all the challenges of recruiting and retaining employees in public health, Katherine reasons that being sensitive to this new generation should be an easier one to tackle. Katherine considers taking a proactive approach by implementing a training program for Bill and his managers to discuss the issue. A training program might give managers of all generations the tools to successfully adapt their culture and better incorporate the values of different generations rather than just dismissing them.

Discussion Questions

1. What should be the main objectives of the training program?

2. What would you include in the training curriculum?

3. What multigenerational management challenges are facing the public health sector?

4. Will a training program help address these challenges?

5. How should Katherine implement this training program for managers? How should she deal with resistance?

References

[1] Association of Schools of Public Health. (2008, February). *Confronting the public health workforce crisis: ASPH statement on the public health workforce*. Retrieved from http://www.asph.org/UserFiles/PHWFShortage0208.pdf

[2] Association of State and Territorial Health Officials. (2008). *2007 State public health workforce survey results*. Retrieved from http://www.astho.org/Display/AssetDisplay.aspx?id=500

Case 26 Managing Diversity

CASE CONTRIBUTOR Scott D. Musch

Situation

Jennifer, a supervisor for the food safety division within the health department of a major metropolitan area, wanted to throw her hands up and shout at the next employee who walked through her office door to complain. She had reached her limit in hearing complaints from her staff members about other coworkers in the department. It seemed like every other day a staff member would come into her office and tell her about a coworker making an insensitive comment or not doing their work the way he or she "should." Although Jennifer was sensitive to reports of any activity contributing to a hostile work environment, she started to think that her employees were being too sensitive and intentionally looking out for comments to support their cases. When her employees joined the department, they participated in diversity training as part of their orientation session, but the lessons they learned seemed to have dissipated.

Supervising a diverse team of employees has its rewards and challenges. Jennifer appreciated the wide range of perspectives and views on public health concerns. The overall staff at the health department was, what Jennifer liked to call, truly cosmopolitan. The staff was reflective of the diversity of the metropolitan area. In Jennifer's department, the cultural diversity was even more pronounced. Jennifer supervised the program responsible for monitoring food service workers and inspecting community restaurants for food safety and health violations. The diversity of her workforce was absolutely necessary to interact successfully with the multicultural restaurant workers within the city. Her employees' diversity contributed greatly to the success of the food safety division.

Jennifer had recently selected a group of her employees to work on a team to evaluate new policies and procedures for restaurant and food safety inspection. She felt the policies and procedures team would give coworkers a better opportunity to get to know each other and improve their working relationships. The objective of the team was to standardize a set of restaurant policies among different counties within the greater metropolitan area. The team needed to discuss which policies worked and which didn't, and then agree on a set of recommendations. The work would require team members to share their cultural perspectives of the food and restaurant practices within the city. Selecting the team was a challenge, as Jennifer wanted to make sure members represented the city's diverse ethnic communities. The final team included Meihui, a Chinese woman; Manuel, a Catholic Hispanic Latino; Susan, a Caucasian lesbian; Knitasha, an African American who was a recent hire from a public health school graduate program; Tom, an Indian who was a veteran with the department and near retirement; and Alima, a female Sunni Muslim. Since inception, the team has been dysfunctional. Certain team members refuse to speak directly to other members. Members make insensitive comments to others, leading to arguments and members storming out of meetings. Other members are completely silent and don't participate during meetings. The animosity between team members has bled over into the general atmosphere of the department, contributing to the increased frequency of complaints arriving at Jennifer's office door.

Background

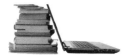

Many managers feel unprepared to lead departments and project teams that comprise diverse individuals of different cultures, ethnic backgrounds, educational levels, ages, genders, sexual orientations, religions, and other heterogeneous mixes. This discomfort can manifest in a lack of understanding and recognition of the competencies necessary to manage a diverse workforce and project teams. The result can be a dysfunctional work environment, with workers becoming less productive, motivated, and easily offended. Low satisfaction levels can increase employee turnover and lead to formal complaints against coworkers, contributing to hostility and suspicion. Managers need to proactively refine and improve their techniques to recognize diversity and improve the overall climate and encourage cooperation. Enhanced skills are required not only to manage a diverse workforce, but to lead productive teams that comprise diverse members.

Effective teamwork offers obvious benefits to team members, including a chance to be creative and share ideas, an opportunity to build stronger working relationships with colleagues, an opportunity to learn new skills or enhance existing ones, among many others. The satisfaction gained from working in teams and creating a collective work productive can be very rewarding. Facilitating and managing a team, however, requires education and experience. Most teams go through four development stages before they become productive, as identified by Bruce W. Tuckman: forming, storming, norming, and performing.[1] The stages can be cyclical and individual team members may be at different stages than other team members. The project manager needs to lead the group through these four stages and keep the members focused on their objective. Incorporating additional levels of diversity into the mix of a team places greater responsibility on the project manager to effectively facilitate the team and root out underlying hostility and insensitivity.

Next Steps

Jennifer is growing increasingly concerned that the team will not succeed in meeting its objectives. Moreover, she is upset that many of her employees seem to be contributing, directly or indirectly, to the heightened level of animosity toward each other in the department. Her department and the policies and procedures team have become dysfunctional. If this continues, her boss and other supervisors at the health department are going to think she is not capable of managing and she may lose her job.

Discussion Questions

1. How would you handle this situation?

2. How could Jennifer manage diversity more effectively in the department?

3. What steps should be taken to reduce the animosity within the department?

4. How would you facilitate the policies and procedures team and get it back on track?

5. Create a cross-cultural sensitivity training program, using the current team members as the audience, to serve as a tool for career development.

Reference

[1] Tuckman, B. W. (1965). Developmental sequence in small groups. *Psychological Bulletin, 63*, 384–399.

Case 27

Broken Promises

CASE CONTRIBUTOR James A. Johnson

Situation

The Department of Psychiatry at Wintergreen University Hospital was originally organized and managed under a traditional, centralized hospital organizational structure.[1] It was later shifted to a quasi-decentralized management system in which operating responsibilities and financial accountability were self-contained within the Department of Psychiatry. Additionally, the department expanded its program by creating the Greenbay Institute of Psychiatry ("Institute") to integrate the new decentralized management system into its triadic purpose of excellence in clinical care, teaching, and research. During the period of preparation for the move to the Institute, management and organization processes were developed but not fully implemented. After development of the Institute, a new facility was built on the grounds of Wintergreen University Hospital to contain nearly all the operations of the Institute and provide inpatient and outpatient care.

Eight months before the move to the Institute, the newly appointed director of nursing, Laura, a Doctor of Nursing Science (DSN), began to hold weekly nursing staff meetings to involve employees in the decision-making process, in anticipation of expanding the role and responsibilities of the nursing staff at the Institute. She indicated that the nursing staff would be able to plan and implement new programs for patients and would receive recognition for their endeavors. She also mentioned that they would have the opportunity to become more involved with the interdisciplinary team approach in the clinical process, could develop new scheduling methods, and would receive more benefits. As the nursing staff became active in this decision-making process by pooling ideas and suggestions, formulating programs, developing a self-scheduling plan, and creating attractive job satisfaction alternatives, their enthusiasm, motivation, and productivity increased.

Four months after the move to the new facility, staff morale plummeted. Nursing staff were informed that the patient census would increase and patient activity would be intensified immediately, but no additional staff would be hired. The local newspaper, the *Wintergreen Chronicle*, disclosed that the newly opened Institute posted an operating debt in excess of one million dollars. Management structure evolved into a formalized hierarchy in which the director of nursing was no longer directly involved with the proposed initiatives, and mid-level management now had control over staff needs. Six months after the move, the nursing staff attrition rate was dramatically high. In fact, the number of FTEs (full-time equivalents) reached a critical low and the Institute was dependent on nursing agencies and university students to provide patient care.

Next Steps

Three months following this stressful period, Laura made a rare appearance at a staff meeting to welcome new nursing staff to the Institute. She described the Institute's ongoing process of evaluating unit needs and changes to implement one of the best psychiatric hospitals in the country. She added that those nursing employees who had resigned "were not flexible and didn't want to work hard." The few remaining original nursing staff of Wintergreen University Hospital who were present noted her statement with raised eyebrows.

Discussion Questions

1. What are the major problems in this situation?

2. How could Laura have handled the situation differently?

3. Discuss the implications of changing from a decentralized to a centralized, hierarchical management structure.

4. What should the nurses do?

Reference

[1] Kilpatrick, A. O., & Johnson, J. A. (1999). *Human resources and organizational behavior: Cases in health services management*. Chicago: Health Administration Press.

Case 28   Sick Building Syndrome

CASE CONTRIBUTOR Scott D. Musch

Situation

Mary hung up the phone and sighed. Larry, the building supervisor, was furious and he vented his emotions to Mary. Larry had just spoken with a project officer from the National Institute for Occupational Safety and Health (NIOSH). The project officer reported that a Health Hazard Evaluation (HHE) request was made by an employee of one of his corporate tenants and the officer wanted to arrange a site visit. NIOSH, a part of the Centers for Disease Control and Prevention (CDC) in the Department of Health and Human Services, is responsible for assuring safe and healthy working conditions. Larry wanted to know which one of Mary's employees had contacted NIOSH and why. He was upset that he was not informed about this ahead of time. His company had completed the renovation of the building and there should not be any health hazards. In addition, if word leaked out about an inspection, he might have trouble leasing the other vacant floors, not to mention the reputational damage with current tenants. Who would want to lease office space in a building being investigated by NIOSH? Mary had listened patiently while Larry vented. She didn't know who contacted NIOSH, and even if she did, she definitely wouldn't share it with Larry.

Mary was the human resources director of Triade Billing Services, a medical billing and claims processing company. Triade was a rapidly growing company with an expanding workforce. The company was headquartered in a large office building in downtown Atlanta and had occupied the building for five years. The office building was constructed in the mid-1990s, but the floors were recently renovated within the last year. The renovation went well and the employees seemed happy with the updated accommodations. Given the nature of the business, the floor layout consisted of closely arranged desk cubicles with computer terminals and other electronic equipment. The office was not unlike most business offices in downtown Atlanta. Mary thought the office space was suitable for employees, though employees occasionally complained of headaches and dry eyes. Everyone blamed the bad air and lighting. Given the nature of their work—long hours in front of computer terminals—Mary felt the problem was most likely due to the glare on their computer screens. However, as the complaints persisted, she contacted Larry to evaluate the fluorescent lights on the floor. After some evaluation, Larry reluctantly agreed to change the power of the lights and within days, the headaches disappeared.

Mary thought this might be the end of the complaints and for the most part, it was. However, a few employees continued to express concerns over the quality of the air in the office. Mary noted that absenteeism due to sick days had gradually trended up over the last year for several employees. One employee in particular concerned her. Doug had recently come down with a chronic breathing problem. He had seen a doctor who thought it might be the onset of asthma, but was unable to determine a direct cause. Doug was convinced that it was building-related asthma and he was not shy sharing his concerns with his fellow workers. Mary, on the other hand, was skeptical. However, she witnessed Doug growing increasingly frustrated at work due to his illness and discomfort. He started to call in sick more often which had been unlike him in the past. There were other employees who reported similar problems but none to the same extent.

Background

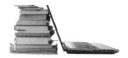

Sick building syndrome (SBS) is a situation in which building occupants experience health symptoms as a result of time spent in a specific building and the illness cannot be traced to a specific cause. Another condition, building-related illness (BRI), is a situation in which the symptoms of an illness can be identified and directly attributed to building contaminants. For instance, BRIs have traceable causes, such as the spread of a virus throughout an office, allergies or asthma due to dust or mold in the workplace, or cancer caused by asbestos or other chemicals. Experts differ in their opinions on the causes of SBS, as to whether it is due to poor indoor air quality from inadequate ventilation, other pollutants, or even work-related stress. Complaints of SBS appear more often in newer, energy efficient buildings where windows are sealed shut and there is limited circulation of outside air. Although experts differ on the causes, they recognize SBS as a serious problem for employees who are suffering with real symptoms and employers who are losing billions of dollars each year in lost productivity.

Next Steps

Mary realized that Doug was likely the employee who contacted NIOSH, probably out of frustration. She wished Doug would have approached her first, but would she have recognized that the work environment may be to blame? She might have tried to convince Larry to run some tests, but given Larry's negative reaction to changing the fluorescent lights, she knew how he would have reacted. The NIOSH project officer is scheduled to visit the building next week to begin the HHE. The evaluation could take several months to a year. In the meantime, Mary, Larry, and Doug will just have to wait.

Discussion Questions

1. How should the NIOSH project officer interact with a skeptical Mary, a disgruntled Larry, and a sick Doug?

2. Did Doug do anything wrong in contacting NIOSH to request an HHE?

3. Can Mary reprimand Doug for contacting NIOSH?

4. What should Mary have done once employees complained of SBS at their workplace?

Case 29

Don't Ask, But Tell

CASE CONTRIBUTOR Scott D. Musch

Situation

The Company Commander, Captain Ronald, listened to the report from the emergency room (ER) physician on the phone. One of his unit members, Army Specialist (SPC) Garrett, was in observation at the Military Treatment Facility (MTF) on the MOB Station for severe injuries. The physician relayed the specific details of the situation. After completing the day's premobilization training and having dinner, SPC Garrett reported to his barracks around 2000 hours (8 p.m.). At 2200 hours (10 p.m.), he came to the MTF dazed and bleeding and was immediately assessed by a medical technician. The medical evaluation intake showed that SPC Garrett suffered contusions, lacerations, and abrasions to his head and torso. In explaining the cause of his injuries, the patient stated that he "fell down" in the barracks. However, his injuries were inconsistent with a fall, and the medic suspected that he had been beaten, and possibly kicked. The medic reported the incident to the ER physician on call who further evaluated the patient. Given the seriousness of the injuries, the physician recommended that SPC Garrett remain under observation for several days as he suspected possible mTBI (mild traumatic brain injury), due to blows to SPC Garrett's head.

Captain (CPT) Ronald absorbed the report. While at first he was shocked by the news, he later realized there had been early signs of escalating aggression. There had been an increasing level of animosity directed toward SPC Garrett by several of his fellow unit members throughout that week's training sessions. SPC Garrett was a good soldier. He was disciplined, physically fit, and technically competent. However, he was more reserved than the other men and as a result seemed to be a bit of an outsider. Some of the other unit members fed on this, and regularly taunted him, including making off-handed remarks about him being gay, or "having sugar in the blood." The taunting escalated after news of the repeal of the Don't Ask, Don't Tell (DADT) policy. While CPT Ronald was aware of the remarks, he generally dismissed them as they didn't rise to the level that warranted any action. He realized now that a few of his men in Charlie company resented the repeal of DADT, and they might have acted out. The company was preparing for an extended mobilization in the AOR (area of responsibility), and CPT Ronald knew he had several decisions to make regarding this potential violation of Uniform Code of Military Justice (UCMJ) against SPC Garrett.

Background

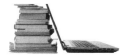

The ban on gay service members dates back to 1950 when the U.S. Congress passed the UCMJ, which established basic policies, discharge procedures, and appeal channels for the disposition of homosexual service members. In January 1981, President Reagan issued Defense Directive 1332.14, which directed the Department of Defense to discharge any gay, lesbian, or bisexual service members pursuant to the UCMJ, declaring homosexuality incompatible with military service. In 1993, in his first year in office, President Clinton called for legislation to end the ban and allow all citizens to serve in the military regardless of sexual orientation. In response, Congress inserted text into the Defense Authorization Act for Fiscal Year 1994, passed in December 1993, requiring the military to abide by regulations essentially identical to the 1982 absolute ban policy (10 U.S.C. § 654). In response, President Clinton issued Defense Directive 1304.26 as an enforcement guideline for the law, which became known as "Don't Ask, Don't Tell." The Defense Directive served as an enforcement policy mandating that military officials not ask about or require members to reveal their sexual orientation, that members may be discharged for claiming to be homosexual or having an intent to engage in homosexual activities, and that military officials are not to pursue rumors about the sexual orientation of the service members or condone harassment or violence against service members for any reason.

In December 2010, the U.S. Congress passed the Don't Ask, Don't Tell Repeal Act of 2010 ending the ban on gay service members. Prior to the repeal taking effect, the President, Secretary of Defense, and Chairman of the Joint Chiefs of Staff had to certify to Congress that the Department of Defense was prepared to implement the repeal and that in doing so there would be no harm to military readiness, military effectiveness, unit cohesion, and recruiting and retention of the Armed Forces. The repeal took effect 60 days after Congress received the certification. Upon passage of the new law, Robert M. Gates, then Secretary of Defense, noted that "successful implementation will depend upon strong leadership, a clear message and proactive education throughout the force."[1]

Next Steps

CPT Ronald planned to visit SPC Garrett in the MTF the next day and press him for the names of the men he suspected were involved in the incident. Once he got their names he would arrange through the Security Forces to handle the interrogation. While an established military justice protocol was in place to deal with this type of situation, CPT Ronald was more concerned about how to defuse any potential for further violence within his unit. He couldn't have more of his unit members heading to the MTF with injuries from altercations or mental health issues. The repeal of DADT was a sensitive topic for some members, and the incident with SPC Garrett may affect unit cohesion. He could not risk any division on the battlefield. Above the individual health and safety concerns of his unit members, he was concerned that the policy might impact the Battle Buddy system that has been an essential part of the military in a deployed environment. CPT Ronald recognized that he needed to send a clear message to his company to defuse any conflict and strengthen the cohesion of his unit.

Discussion Questions

1. What message should CPT Ronald deliver to his unit in response to the incident with SPC Garrett?

2. How did the military's policy on homosexuality imperil the health of service members, the military, and the country (consider undiagnosed STDs, medical history intake, mental health)?

3. What implications will the repeal of DADT have on the health of services members and the community at large?

Reference

[1] Wong, S. (2010, December 18). "Don't ask" repeal wins final passage. *Politico*. Retrieved from http://www.politico.com/news/stories/1210/46576.html

Case 30 — Top Ten U.S. Public Health Achievements

CASE CONTRIBUTOR **Scott D. Musch**

Situation

Ethan is the training coordinator for a large state public health agency in the Northwest. He is in the process of preparing the new employee orientation program for the agency. The objectives of the program are to provide a general overview of the department, services offered, and administrative policies and procedures to efficiently prepare the employees for their job duties. Among the standard topics included in the orientation session will be the requirements of confidentiality surrounding health services to ensure full compliance with the law as well as other functional responsibilities.

One of the goals of the agency's workforce recruiting program has been to focus on hiring qualified workers for the public health system overall and not just for individual programs and agencies. This recruitment strategy has been successful in attracting professionals from the business field and other areas outside of public health. The pipeline of new recruits will help ensure an adequate supply of professionals for the agency to eliminate the critical public health workforce shortage experienced by many employers within the field.

As many of the agency's new employees will come from positions outside of the field, Ethan believes that the orientation program should contain a session or workshop on the 10 greatest achievements in U.S. public health over the last century. He hopes that by including this instruction in the program new employees will develop a base public health competence, enabling them to understand the crucial role public health has played in all aspects of society. The workshop will provide an opportunity for new employees to learn the significance and scope of public health initiatives as well as to broaden their awareness of the needs and challenges within the field.

Background

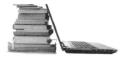

In 1999, the Centers for Disease Control and Prevention (CDC) prepared a list of the notable public health achievements that occurred during the 20th century (Table 30–1). The choices were based on the opportunity for prevention and the impact on death, illness, and disability in the United States. The list was not ranked by order of importance.

Table 30–1 Ten Great Public Health Achievements in the U.S. (1900–1999)

- Vaccination
- Motor vehicle safety
- Safer workplaces
- Control of infectious diseases
- Decline in deaths from coronary heart disease and stroke
- Safer and healthier foods
- Healthier mothers and babies
- Family planning
- Fluoridation of drinking water
- Recognition of tobacco use as a health hazard

Source: *"Ten Great Public Health Achievements—United States, 1900–1999," Centers for Disease Control and Prevention,* Morbidity and Mortality Weekly Report, 48*(12), pp. 241–243.*[1]

Next Steps

To develop the workshop, Ethan has arranged for several health analysts in the agency to prepare background research on each of the topics on the list. Ethan wants the session to be highly informative so the new employees will appreciate these contributions of public health and understand their effect on the health of persons in the United States.

Discussion Questions

1. If you were the training coordinator, how would you design the workshop to meet the goals of the agency?

2. How will understanding the history help new professionals develop a base competence in public health and help their career development?

3. What other accomplishments could have been selected for the list?

Reference

[1] Centers for Disease Control and Prevention. (1999, April 2). Ten Great Public Health Achievements – United States, 1900–1999. *Morbidity and Mortality Weekly Report, 48*(12), 241–243. Retrieved from http://www.cdc.gov/mmwr/preview/mmwrhtml/00056796.htm

Case 31

Tuberculosis in the Workplace

CASE CONTRIBUTORS Domingo J. Navarro and Scott D. Musch

Situation

Dominic, the communicable disease program manager for the Tuberculosis and Hansen Disease Program at a local health department, received a letter from the Human Resources (HR) office regarding an employee of the organization. The HR department received a complaint from a supervisor who was concerned that an employee of his may be transmitting a communicable disease to others at her work. The supervisor wanted to have all the immediate employees checked for tuberculosis (TB) as well as the supervisor's family.

Gabriela was an employee and coworker in the local health department. She worked for one of the programs that provided medical transportation to elderly, disabled, and young children. She had been working for many years and was a very dedicated employee. One day she did not come to work as she had gotten sick and had to be hospitalized. No one at her office knew her situation except for her immediate supervisor and the local health department director. After a few weeks she returned to work and had been scheduled to go to one of the public health clinics based on a referral by her private physician. Gabriela was referred to a TB outpatient clinic. She was seen by a TB physician who placed her on treatment for an active disease.

On one of those clinic visits, Dominic saw her and recognized her as his coworker. He asked how she was doing and she said she was not feeling well, but that she was glad to be out of the hospital. She mentioned that she had been admitted to a private hospital due to a cough that would not go away and she had some fever. When she showed up to the emergency room, she was admitted to the hospital for observation. She showed the medications to Dominic, he told her that she should take the medications as they would be important for her to get cured for her TB. She mentioned to him that she didn't feel sick and that the medications made her nauseous and sick. A few weeks later she went back to work and she mentioned to Dominic that her husband had been tested and that his TB test was negative. She also mentioned that he was cleared of tuberculosis. In their conversation, she mentioned that her medications were making her feel very lethargic and tired and that she did not feel well, yet she continued to go to work.

Background

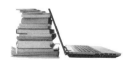

Tuberculosis or TB (short for *mycobacterium tuberculosis*) is one of the oldest known diseases to afflict humans and affects nearly one third of the world's population. It affects individuals in many parts of the world who are living in crowded conditions and in poverty. TB is a common and often deadly infectious disease caused by the TB germ passed from human to human. TB usually attacks the lungs but can also affect other parts of the body. The disease is transmitted through the air when people who have the disease cough, sneeze, or sing. Individuals who spend over six to eight hours daily around a contagious TB case can inhale the germ and become infected. Signs and symptoms of TB are a cough with many weeks' duration, weight loss, fatigue, night sweats, and fever.

TB is treatable and if caught in time, it can be cured. Individuals who are treated early become noncontagious and can return to work within three or four weeks after beginning their anti-TB medications. Additional tests, such as a sputum collection, are done to get reports on identifying whether the germ is still active or not. An individual is noncontagious when his or her culture or laboratory results on the sputum are negative on three separate consecutive collection dates. Laboratory results on sputa and cultures are very important for the clinician treating a TB case. The findings on x-rays also are important to demonstrate improvement and show that no cavitations from the bacteria are occurring when compared to previous chest x-rays.

Next Steps

Dominic was concerned about what his fellow employees at the local health department office were discussing about a TB case in their midst. In a conversation with the TB physician at the outpatient clinic, Dominic heard some interesting observations regarding some patients who had been referred to the clinic. The doctor said that he had been receiving quite a few referrals on various individuals with identical admission dates at the same private hospital from within the local health department jurisdiction. These patients had all been diagnosed with active TB. In addition, he mentioned that five additional patients referred to the clinic showed no abnormalities in their x-rays as well as no symptoms. Interestingly, the physician stated that they all seemed fine. Dominic and the physician discussed the smear and culture identification in all five patients as having grown tuberculosis. The similarity and the culture results on all five patients, including Gabriela, appeared to be a public health concern. Gabriela had been admitted to the hospital around the same time as the other patients who had been scheduled to have their follow-up at the TB outpatient clinic. Dominic started to think TB testing should be done on all immediate employees and their families at the department.

Discussion Questions

1. Should all of Gabriella's coworkers and supervisor and the supervisor's family be tested?

2. Was Gabriela a threat to coworkers after being diagnosed with TB?

3. What should the HR department have done upon receiving the complaint from the supervisor?

4. How should the HR department handle this type of complaint?

5. What actions should Dominic and the TB physician have taken once numerous TB referrals were being sent to the outpatient clinic? Could there have been a possible laboratory reporting error?

6. Has a HIPAA violation or breach of information occurred in the department?

Case 32 | Zero Tolerance for Smoking

CASE CONTRIBUTOR Scott D. Musch

Situation

Theresa arrived early in the office. As supervisor of Mandover Health Clinic, a large community health center (CHC) in a suburb of Chicago, she had a full agenda planned for the day. However, she couldn't stop thinking about what she witnessed the previous evening. After work she had taken her family to the Olive Garden restaurant for dinner. As she was walking into the restaurant, she noticed out of the corner of her eye one of her employees, Hanna, smoking in the parking lot. Theresa was dismayed—what a surprising and disappointing sight. She didn't expect to see any of her employees smoking, not to mention one of her most senior ones. Hanna was well liked by the staff at Mandover. She performed her duties well at the clinic and the rest of the staff often sought her out for advice. However, by smoking Hanna was setting a poor example for the organization and even more so as a seasoned health professional.

The Mandover Health Clinic is a smoke-free workplace as required by the Smoke Free Illinois Act that went into effect in 2008. The act prohibits smoking in a public place or place of employment. Employees who smoke at a workplace can be fired for violating the law. Theresa has not seen any employees smoking outside the building so she assumed, incorrectly of course, that none of her employees smoked. Moreover, she expected that as public health workers they would know the dangers of smoking and would naturally choose not to smoke. The more Theresa thought about the situation, the more upset she became. Mandover offers a smoking cessation program to new employees and she thought the program was successful. Theresa wondered how many other employees might be smoking off-duty. Theresa felt somewhat embarrassed thinking about her public health employees smoking behind her back. Don't they realize that smoking increases health insurance premiums, not to mention it reflects badly on the image of Mandover as a community health clinic?

Background

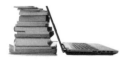

More companies are adopting zero-tolerance smoking policies that prohibit employees from smoking in their private lives. Employers are firing employees who fail to quit smoking after a period of time and are even banning the hiring of people who smoke. The adoption of zero-tolerance policies has accompanied the enactment of smoke-free work and public places laws by states, municipalities, and companies. Twenty-four U.S. states and commonwealths now have 100% smoke-free laws that prohibit smoking in all workplaces, restaurants, and bars.[1]

Employers support these policies as a means to curb rising healthcare costs. However, there may be a more idealistic objective. Healthcare companies, including public health agencies, may well consider the example they are setting by accepting employees who smoke despite the knowledge of the inherent health risks of such behavior. The thinking goes that if an employee of a healthcare company who should know the health consequences can't be responsible enough not to smoke, then who can be? The World Health Organization (WHO) has set an illustrative policy. According to the WHO's Smoking and Tobacco Use Policy, the organization will not recruit smokers or other tobacco users. The policy states that "In the case of tobacco, the importance for WHO not to be seen as 'normalizing' tobacco use also warrants consideration in the Organization's recruitment policy" and "The Organization has a responsibility to ensure that this is reflected in all its work, including in its recruitment practices and in the image projected by the Organization and its staff members."[2]

Next Steps

Theresa debated whether to set a strict example of Hanna by showing that smoking would not be tolerated by any employee at Mandover. She had a range of options from asking employees to sign a pledge not to smoke as a condition of employment to mandating random testing. If an employee chose not to take a test or the test came back positive, then their employment would be terminated. She wondered whether there would be much resistance in implementing such programs, particularly considering they worked for a health clinic. However, first she needed to decide what action to take with Hanna. She could ask Hanna to participate in the clinic's anti-smoking program, but if she refused, Theresa may have to let her go.

Discussion Questions

1. What would you do if you were the supervisor faced with this situation?

2. Should an employer fire an employee who refuses to stop smoking?

3. What human resources policies are available to encourage employees to quit smoking?

4. What do you think of the WHO's Smoking and Tobacco Use Policy? Should a healthcare organization, in its role as an employer, observe a higher standard with respect to specific health behaviors that are deemed acceptable for its employees?

References

[1] American Nonsmokers' Rights Foundation. (2011, January 2). U.S. 100% Smokefree laws in workplaces and restaurants and bars. Retrieved from http://www.no-smoke.org/pdf/WRBLawsMap.pdf

[2] World Health Organization. (2008, September). WHO policy on non-recruitment of smokers or other tobacco users: Frequently asked questions. Retrieved from the World Health Organization at http://www.who.int/employment/FAQs_smoking_English.pdf

Case 33 — Ethiopia's Struggle with Resource Management

CASE CONTRIBUTOR **David J. Ranney**

Situation

Ethiopia's national healthcare system is both mismanaged and donor dependent. The country's leadership, fearful of losing either the outside supplies or aid, has adopted a "we'll take whatever you give us" attitude. Problematic to this approach is what you receive is seldom what you need. The end results are hospital warehouses filled with unusable supplies (from medications to gloves to operating equipment) and lines of patients without their medications and supplies. To fix this, Ethiopian leadership needs to review its "open door policy" of accepting anything and everything and requesting that if a donor wants to give something, it must be something the nation can use. This will require not only strong leadership but, more importantly, a real understanding of what the nation needs.

As a member of the Yale-Clinton Foundation sponsored Ethiopia Hospital Management Initiative (EHMI), David and a group of management fellows went to Ethiopia to coach and mentor senior-level hospital administrators on decision-making tools, project design, implementation, and follow-up. David's background in logistics and process improvement taught him that sweeping change is never easy. He realized at the start that taking on the challenge of a bottom-up, national change would challenge both his academic and professional training.

Within his assigned region of Amhara (located in the central highlands of Ethiopia), David was charged with tackling the issues of addressing and fixing a broken pharmacy system and a complete overhaul of the supply chain. His responsibilities included training the administration on lean and six sigma tools (business management/waste reduction tools that help improve an organization's output quality by removing defects and wasteful processes) to helping design policies and procedures for smooth material flows. At the top of David's task list was to listen and watch the people, pay attention to how processes work (or not), and empower the staff to come up with ideas for improving the hospital.

Background

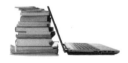

"Ethiopia is the oldest independent country in Africa and one of the oldest in the world."[1] In 1993, Ethiopia released its 20-year, multisector health policy strategic plan that "proposes realistic goals and the means for attaining them based on the fundamental principles that health, constituting physical, mental and social well-being, is a prerequisite for the enjoyment of life and for optimal productivity."[2]

The Yale-Clinton Foundation is a collaboration between Yale University and the William J. Clinton Foundation HIV/AIDS Initiative (CHAI). The Clinton Foundation states, "CHAI is a global health organization committed to strengthening integrated health systems in the developing world and expanding access to care and treatment for HIV/AIDS, malaria, and tuberculosis."[3]

The EHMI is a project developed and sponsored by the Yale-Clinton Foundation with an objective to bring management and leadership theory into practice. The goal of EHMI can be expressed best by the Ethiopian Minister of Health, Dr. Tedros Adhanom Ghebeysus, in a speech he gave to the fellows shortly after landing in Ethiopia: "I don't care if you make mistakes . . . I just want you to help make change." Dr. Elizabeth Bradley, project leader for Yale University School of Public Health, expanded on Dr. Tedros' plea: "The goal of the EHMI is to enhance the management capacity of hospitals in Ethiopia using a systems-based approach. This will be achieved by replicating improved management systems that advance patient care and outcomes in hospitals throughout the country."[4]

David was part of a team assigned to the Felege Hiwot Regional Referral Hospital (FHRRH) in Bahir Dar, Ethiopia. The hospital leadership was primarily the responsibility of the clinical administrator/Chief of Staff, Dr. Bader (a pediatric surgeon by trade). Assisting Dr. Bader on daily tasks was the general administrator, Mr. Simachew. The hospital pharmacist was in charge of ordering and warehousing both medical and non-medical supplies.

David focused on three specific projects while at FHRRH:

- Pharmacy Warehouse. There is a saying in the warehouse world, "If you can't find it, you don't have it." The warehouse at FHRRH was in chaos and it was common practice for a physician to be told that medication was not on-hand only to find it at a later point.
- Medical Library. Having a dedicated place for medical research (books, Internet access, quiet space) is a necessary requirement for a hospital. Upon arrival at FHRRH, there was no space for a library and no plan for acquiring the needed supplies.
- Pharmacy Formulary. If the pharmacist's order is different from what the physician prescribed, the patient suffers. Having a formulary on-hand tells the provider what the pharmacy carries and recommends for specific illnesses. To be acceptable, the formulary must be a combined effort of both providers and pharmacy staff.

Next Steps

David's challenges were primarily employee-centric involving creating excitement for change, encouraging employees to generate their own ideas, establishing buy-in, and empowering employees to take control of a process. Other challenges included opening lines of communication and trust between the chief pharmacist/supply officer and physicians as well as convincing the hospital chief of staff to give his employees more room.

The employee challenges proved most difficult for two main reasons: the staff was comfortable with leaving "well enough alone" and the salary structure stifled any desire to take on more responsibility. Opening lines of communication and creating a level of trust between the pharmacy and providers proved to be an exercise of ongoing discussion. The more often each side got together and talked, the more comfortable they became with each other. Once the pharmacist knew he was being taken seriously, he was much more willing and able to confront the providers on matters related to medication administration and supply availability and use.

The leadership of the Ethiopian national health system continues to address the challenges it now faces. There is a need for outside assistance, but not necessarily in the form of consultant reports. Ethiopians recognize they need people with the knowledge and desire to jump in and teach them. As David learned, the people will learn.

Discussion Questions

1. Public health agencies rely on donors and in some cases, such as in Ethiopia, may become "donor dependent." How should public health leaders manage this issue, particularly when it involves wasting supplies?

2. In addressing a national public health infrastructure, how is a ground-up approach more effective than a top-down approach?

3. In working with a team tasked with improving the public health system for a less-developed country such as Ethiopia, how might you frame the challenge? How do you address the issue of overwhelmed resources?

4. In Ethiopia, patients will often show up at agencies in a poor state. Although you might be tempted when asked to intervene and offer assistance (such as money, taxi fare), why should you resist?

5. As a public health worker in a foreign country, what is the danger of saying "Back in the States, we do it this way?"

References

[1] Central Intelligence Agency. (2011, January 12). *The world factbook: Africa: Ethiopia* (Fact Sheet). Retrieved from CIA – The World Factbook at https://www.cia.gov/library/publications/the-world-factbook

[2] Federal Ministry of Health, Ethiopia. (1993). *Health policy of the transitional government of Ethiopia: September 1993*. Retrieved from Ethiomedic at www.ethiomedic.com/index.php/national-guidelines/file/358-healthpolicyofthetransitionalgovernmentofethiopiasept1993.html?start=15

[3] William J. Clinton Foundation. (2011). *Treating HIV/AIDS and malaria: Clinton health access initiative*. Retrieved from http://www.clintonfoundation.org/what-we-do/clinton-health-access-initiative

[4] Yale School of Public Health and William J. Clinton Foundation. (2007). *Blueprint for hospital management in Ethiopia* (Policy Brief). Retrieved from Yale University at http://publichealth.yale.edu

Case 34 | The Family Health Initiative

CASE CONTRIBUTOR Victor D. Weeden

Situation

Lieutenant Colonel James White is the chief of medical services for an overseas military treatment facility. During the past year, he has directed the implementation of a new primary care model at a United States Air Force (USAF) Hospital in Europe. His task is to transform the delivery of family health care by implementing the Air Force Medical Service (AFMS) Family Health Initiative (FHI). The FHI is the AFMS implementation model for the patient-centered medical home (PCMH). The PCMH was historically used in the civilian healthcare sector and more recently in the Military Health System. The FHI implementation was completed on schedule at the AFMS hospital without major disruption to medical service operations. However, Lieutenant Colonel White is concerned about the long-term sustainability of the FHI transformation and energizing medical facility leadership and staff to maintain the continuous improvement gains realized.

The foundation of the PCMH model is the physician-led team. Lieutenant Colonel White's supervisors have charged him with directing the transformation of family health care by leading change and cultivating partnership at all levels. In turn, the physician leaders at each medical facility must embrace the PCMH vision and set the tone for success. Lieutenant Colonel White must strategically guide and support the physician leaders to ensure necessary resources are available and appropriately aligned in the organization.[1] In addition, physician leaders must provide mentorship to clinical staff and ensure that population health and disease management programs are progressing. Lieutenant Colonel White is thoroughly convinced that the FHI model is appropriate for military family health care and will be successful under the right conditions. However, he is concerned about previous military primary care models that failed for a variety of reasons, including lack of staffing, unrealistic expectations/timelines, inadequate implementation plans, and inappropriate metric indicators.

Background

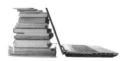

The PCMH model was introduced in 1967 by the American Academy of Pediatrics (AAP) to improve health outcomes for patients with chronic conditions. PCMH is also endorsed by the American Academy of Family Physicians and American College of Physicians.[1] PCMH has been associated with improved medical outcomes and provides an integrated team approach to delivering health care. The professional literature indicates that PCMH can have a significant positive impact on controlling healthcare costs, reducing emergency room demand, enhancing patient satisfaction, and decreasing physician turnover.

In turn, the FHI is designed to provide high-quality population-based health care within a productive and rewarding practice environment. The keys to its success include maximizing patient involvement, optimizing use of the entire healthcare team, increasing continuity between staff and patients, and maximizing team communication.[2] The FHI integrates family primary care activities with population disease management, case management, and a prevention focus. The FHI was developed and introduced to address patient concerns about appointment availability, lack of provider continuity, and a quality healthcare experience that could be enhanced through strong provider-patient relationships. The FHI was also developed to address staff concerns such as past inability to build continuity with patients, inadequate support staff, lack of control over provider practice, and treatment of a poorly assigned patient population that lacks complexity and acuity necessary to practice quality medicine.

Next Steps

Lieutenant Colonel White will be meeting with his team during the next week to conduct a status review and address any staff or patient issues. Certain medical providers and support staff have expressed concern about how FHI will ultimately benefit the healthcare organization and patients. Certain providers have reservations about the availability of support staff, quality of decision making between clinical teams, turnover of medical staff due to military commitments, and whether the FHI will actually improve the health of the population. In addition, providers expressed reservations about the effectiveness of integrated teams in selecting the appropriate patient population and managing their health care in the most effective manner possible. The medical facility executive team also requested additional guidance on the best practices available to market FHI to medical providers, support staff, and patient population. This is a crucial period in FHI implementation for the medical facility and may determine the success or failure of the program. Lieutenant Colonel White must decide how to best advise the executive team to proceed, so they can realize the substantial benefits associated with PCMH and population-based health management.

Discussion Questions

1. What strategies would you recommend to Lieutenant Colonel White to energize the executive leadership and staff toward embracing the PCMH concepts and implementing FHI?

2. How would you advise the staff to market FHI to the patient population and promote its benefits?

3. Explain how you would address the concerns raised by provider staff regarding the effectiveness of integrated teams in population health management.

References

[1] Ediger, M. A. (2011, January). The patient-centered medical home. Briefing given at the Air Force Family Health Initiative Workshop, San Antonio, Texas.

[2] Kosmatka, T. J. (2011, January). Global family health initiative. Briefing given at the Air Force Family Health Initiative Workshop, San Antonio, Texas.

Case 35

The Anti-Vaccination Paradigm

CASE CONTRIBUTOR Scott D. Musch

Situation

Dr. Anne London, chief of immunization at the Franklin County Health Agency, reviewed the reports on her desk on the progress of the immunization program in her county. She was particularly concerned as she studied the reports: the overall rate of vaccine refusal remained low at 2.7% but has continued to climb over the last five years. She wondered if Franklin County was setting itself up for a potential public health issue. Outbreaks were no longer unheard of in the United States, especially when considering the measles outbreak in San Diego in 2008, the *pertussis* (whooping cough) outbreak in California in 2010, and even more troubling, the measles epidemic in Great Britain over the last decade.

Dr. London has seen the websites, blogs, and homemade videos—Mom's Against Vaccine Enforcement, among others—claiming a link between vaccines, particularly MMR (measles, mumps, and rubella) and autism. In implementing the immunization program, Dr. London made sure to emphasize education to dispel such beliefs. She recognized that most parents who refuse vaccines for their children are concerned about possible adverse effects and are skeptical of the government, pharmaceutical industry, and medical community. She could empathize to a degree with these parents, as they are probably acting in good faith and love for their children. After all, she seriously weighs every decision she has to make that may affect her daughter's health. However, don't these parents realize that by failing to immunize their children they place not only their children at a greater risk of disease but the community as a whole?

Background

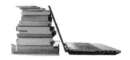

Vaccines have been successful and with that success a new generation of parents in the United States has emerged who have not experienced the terrible effects of polio, measles, whooping cough, and smallpox. Measles outbreaks started to recur in the United States nearly eight years after the virus was declared dead in the United States, largely attributed to a successful vaccination program that began in the 1960s. In 2008, the United States experienced its largest outbreak of measles in more than 10 years affecting 15 states.[1] In 2010, California experienced an outbreak of *pertussis* with more than 4000 reported cases and nine infant deaths linked to the outbreak.[2] These outbreaks have ignited concern over community clusters in which a growing number of parents are intentionally refusing to vaccinate their children. Parents are permitted to do so by signing a personal-beliefs exemption. In the United States, all states require under law children to be properly immunized before attending school. However, exemptions are permitted. In addition to medical exemptions offered in each state, 48 states allow for religious exemptions and 20 states allow personal belief exemptions for daycare and school.[3] Fears that vaccines cause autism, attention deficit hyperactivity disorder (ADHD/ADD), asthma, and allergies are continually fed through viral marketing—websites and blogs purporting vaccination conspiracies—despite the many studies and expert commentary that dispel any scientific link.

The potential seriousness of vaccination noncompliance can be witnessed by looking at the measles epidemic that reemerged in Great Britain over the last decade. After a British medical journal published a study in 1998 in which British researcher Andrew Wakefield suggested that the MMR vaccine triggered autism, vaccination rates in parts of Great Britain fell precipitously, from a national average of 92% in the mid-1990s to 88.4% in 2000, to a low of 75% in some areas of London and Wales.[4] The World Health Organization states that a community needs a vaccination rate of 95% to ensure the herd immunity threshold.[5] Cases of measles have grown annually in Great Britain and Wales as a result of children not getting immunized. (Notably, not only was the Wakefield study retracted in 2010, but another British medical journal, *BMJ,* published an analysis in 2011 that found Wakefield's research to be fraudulent.[6]) Despite the public health consequences, anti-vaccination campaigns still continue in communities within Great Britain and the United States.

Next Steps

Later in the week, Dr. London has a meeting scheduled with her team to review the new immunization program data. After seeing the continuing rise in the rate of vaccine refusals, she plans to ask her team to suggest changes to the immunization program campaign to increase vaccination compliance rates. As chief of immunization at the Franklin County Health Agency, Dr. London wants to be proactive. We need to remain vigilant, Dr. London reflects, and we need to use multiple angles—education, access, and outreach.

Discussion Questions

1. What strategies should the team recommend to Dr. London?

2. How do you deal with parents who refuse to vaccinate their children?

3. As a public health official, should you promote vaccination compliance as a civil responsibility?

4. How do you manage a conflict among individual behavior, organizational behavior, and public health goals?

References

[1] Dunham, W. (2008, July 9). Measles outbreak hits 127 people in 15 states. *Reuters*. Retrieved from http://www.reuters.com/article/idUSN0943743120080709

[2] Mitchell, D. (2010, September 27). Most toddler vaccination rates near national goals but

outbreaks show need for docs to continue educating parents. *AAFP News Now*. Retrieved from http://www.aafp.org/online/en/home/publications/news/news-now/clinical-care-research/20100927toddlervaccs.html

[3] Institute for Vaccine Safety, John Hopkins Bloomberg School of Public Health. (2011, January 6). *Vaccine exemptions*. Retrieved from http://www.vaccinesafety.edu/cc-exem.htm

[4] Laurance, J. (2000, August 8). UK measles outbreak feared after Dublin deaths. *The Independent*. Retrieved from http://www.independent.co.uk/life-style/health-and-families/health-news/uk-measles-outbreak-feared-after-dublin-deaths-710635.html

[5] Georgette, N. (2007). The quantification of the effects of changes in population parameters on the herd immunity threshold. *The Internet Journal of Epidemiology, 5*(1). Retrieved from http://www.ispub.com/ostia/index.php?xmlFilePath=journals/ije/vol5n1/population.xml

[6] Deer, B. (2011, January 8). Secrets of the MMR scare: How the case against the MMR vaccine was fixed. *BMJ, 342*(7788), 77–82. doi: 10.1136/bmj.c5347

Case 36

Collaborative Approach to Diabetes Prevention and Care

CASE CONTRIBUTOR Scott D. Musch

Situation

In 2010, UnitedHealth Group (UHG), a leading health benefits and managed care company (www.unitedhealthgroup.com), announced an innovative new model, the Diabetes Prevention and Control Alliance ("Alliance"), to help prevent and control diabetes, prediabetes, and obesity.[1] The Alliance is anchored by two integrated programs: the Diabetes Prevention Program (DPP) and the Diabetes Control Program (DCP). The DPP is a partnership between the YMCA of the USA (YMCA) and UHG that offers through local community YMCAs a group-based lifestyle intervention for people at high risk of developing diabetes. The YMCA provides lifestyle coaches to help participants learn to eat healthier and increase their physical activity through a 16-session program, with monthly support thereafter to maintain their progress. The YMCA's DPP is based on the Diabetes Prevention Program funded by the National Institutes of Health (NIH) and the CDC.[2] UHG will reimburse YMCAs offering the DPP. The DCP is a partnership between UHG and Walgreens that provides diabetics with access to community-based pharmacists who will provide education and behavioral intervention in the convenient setting of a local pharmacy. Health plan participants whose employers offer the programs and who are identified with diabetes or prediabetes through UHG's screening model are invited to participate voluntarily in the programs at no cost.

Karen, the director of Government Funding, Accountability and Funding at the YMCA, recognizes that the Alliance has the potential to have meaningful systemwide effects on the diabetes epidemic. In particular, the program extends service delivery beyond the traditional physician office setting. The YMCAs and Walgreens have considerable reach and scale, and they increase access to a much larger group of people in the community at high risk for diabetes. For instance, 57% of U.S. households are located within three miles of a YMCA.[3] Reception from local communities in the pilot cities has been generally positive, but there will need to be an education campaign to fully inform qualifying candidates to optimize participation. Karen has been working with the program coordinators within the YMCA and UHG to develop informational campaigns. The YMCA trainers and the community-based pharmacists represent significant access points to increase responsiveness and equity in the system. The YMCA is making the DPP available to everyone who meets the criteria regardless of their health insurance coverage.

Background

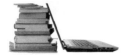

The diabetes epidemic in the United States is accelerating at an alarming rate. According to the CDC, approximately 24 million people or 7.8% of the U.S. population had diabetes in 2007 and another 57 million had prediabetes.[4] By 2020, an estimated 52% of the adult population will have diabetes or prediabetes and more than 90% of those with prediabetes will be unaware of their condition.[5] Private spending, largely borne by employers and employees, is currently estimated at $57 billion a year and is projected to reach nearly $1 trillion in total between 2011 and 2020.[5] The epidemic will have major implications for people's health and healthcare costs, placing a financial strain on families, employers, insurers, states, and the federal government.

Progression to diabetes among those with prediabetes and to complications among those with diabetes is not inevitable. Research from the CDC indicates that two-thirds of all diabetics do not follow their physicians' advice or treatment guidelines on how to manage their disease.[6] People struggle to maintain a healthy lifestyle and often lack knowledge about diabetes and prediabetes conditions. There is substantial evidence that interventions ranging from lifestyle changes to early support for diabetic-related complications can make a meaningful difference in reducing the health and financial toll of diabetes. For instance, research shows that a typical prediabetic person who reduces body weight by 7% through a combination of exercise and caloric restriction can reduce the risk of becoming diabetic by 58%.[7]

Successful interventions will require new approaches outside of medical management of the complications of diabetes, which has been the traditional focus of treatment for the disease. Not only will this require engagement of patients and healthcare providers, but also health insurers if a real meaningful impact is to be made on the epidemic. Employers are increasingly looking to insurers to do more to manage healthcare costs than just collecting premiums and paying providers.[8] With enactment of the new federal healthcare law, insurers will be required to cover people regardless of their medical condition so the financial implications are clear. Despite the benefits of early intervention, until recently no insurance company has paid for evidence-based diabetes prevention and control programs.

The initiative by UHG represents a new paradigm in health care focused on prevention. As indicated in a statement by the chairman of UHG's Center for Health Reform & Modernization, Simon Stevens, there is recognition of the new role health insurers must play in the system: "It will mean a focus not only on the 'flow' of health care consumption, but on managing the 'stock' of population health risk."[5] UHG is using its broad assets in technology, health data, evidence-based medical decision making, and disease management to ensure the dissemination and use of reliable and timely information in the program. UHG, as one of the nation's largest health insurers, is providing the primary source of financing. UHG will cover the services at no charge to plan participants enrolled in employer-provided health insurance plans. The Alliance represents the first time in the United States that a health plan will pay for evidence-based diabetes prevention and control programs.[1] To fortify these efforts, UHG has committed $2.25 million to support the YMCA's healthy-living and obesity prevention initiatives.[9]

Next Steps

Karen is impressed with how the Alliance brings together partners from the private, public, and nonprofit sectors to provide leadership and governance to successfully implement the programs. The YMCA and UHG are slowly rolling out the programs nationally, starting with seven markets in four states: Cincinnati, Columbus, and Dayton, Ohio; Indianapolis, Indiana; Minneapolis and St. Paul, Minnesota; and Phoenix, Arizona. This coordinated approach recognizes that the programs will evolve as they are implemented in different markets. Prevention and control of diabetes in the healthcare system are tightly linked. UHG and employers understand that by engaging individuals to take preventive steps they can decrease the odds of employees moving into higher-cost treatment categories. Participants who regularly follow the programs will receive financial incentives, positive encouragement, and motivation through improved health.

As the benefits become tangible, more employers, employees, and insurers will likely offer similar programs. Reimbursing a community-based organization for delivering prevention and control programs may seem counterintuitive for a profit-oriented company. However, UHG may protect itself in the long run as diabetic patients who do not control their disease could become future liabilities if they change jobs and join employers who are fully insured by UHG. All insurers benefit from healthier members. It is cheaper to give up co-payments and premiums rather than pay for full-blown diabetic disease conditions later. Ultimately, interventions to a system that rely on behavioral modifications are likely to face resistance to change. Although the benefits of prevention and control appear obvious, participation is not assured and insurance coverage for these programs and the financial incentives offered are crucial steps to get more people engaged. Karen recognizes as a relatively new intervention program, both at the YMCA and UHG, the Alliance will face future challenges.

Discussion Questions

1. Discuss how the initiative by the YMCA and UHG represents a new paradigm in health care focused on prevention.

2. What are some of the challenges bringing together partners from the private, public, and nonprofit sectors to successfully implement programs such as the Alliance?

3. How should each organization measure the success of the programs?

4. How are public health program initiatives enhanced by private and public sector partnerships?

5. Do you think a profit-oriented company working with a community-based, nonprofit organization to deliver a public health program is counterintuitive?

6. What issues do you think the partners will face as they slowly roll out the Alliance on a nationwide basis?

References

[1] UnitedHealth Group. (2010, April 14). UnitedHealth Group launches innovative alliance providing free access to programs that help prevent and control diabetes and obesity [Press release]. Retrieved from http://www.unitedhealthgroup.com/newsroom/news.aspx?id=199e50a5-557b-4353-b96d-ff060fba10fc

[2] YMCA of the USA. (2010, April 14). YMCA of the USA, UnitedHealth Group collaboration offers new model for chronic disease prevention [Press release]. Retrieved from http://www.ymca.net/news-releases/20100414-ymca-unitedhealth.html

[3] Vaughan, L. (2010, July 10). The YMCA's Diabetes Prevention Program. Presentation at the Alliance for Health Reform Briefing Co-Sponsored by UnitedHealth Foundation.

[4] U.S. Department of Health and Human Services, Centers for Disease Control and Prevention. (2008). National diabetes fact sheet: General information and national estimates on diabetes in the United States, 2007. Retrieved from http://www.cdc.gov/diabetes/pubs/pdf/ndfs_2007.pdf

[5] UnitedHealth Group. (2010, November). *The United States of diabetes: Challenges and opportunities in the decade ahead* (UnitedHealth Center for Health Reform & Modernization Working Paper 5). Retrieved from http://www.unitedhealthgroup.com/hrm/UNH_WorkingPaper5.pdf

[6] UnitedHealthcare. (2009, January 15). UnitedHealthcare launches first diabetes plan with incentives for preventive care [Press release]. Retrieved from http://www.uhc.com/news_room/2009_news_release_archive/unitedhealthcare_launches_diabetes_plan_with_incentives_for_preventive_care.htm

[7] UnitedHealthcare. (2009, January). Diabetes Health Plan: Fact Sheet January 2009. Retrieved from http://www.uhc.com/live/uhc_com/Assets/Documents/DiabetesHealthPlan.pdf

[8] Abelson, R. (2010, April 13). An insurer's new approach to diabetes. *The New York Times*. Retrieved from http://www.nytimes.com/2010/04/14/health/14diabetes.html?_r=1

[9] UnitedHealth Group. (2010, October 4). UnitedHealth Group pledges $2.25 million to fortify the Y's efforts to prevent obesity and related chronic diseases [Press release]. Retrieved from http://www.unitedhealthgroup.com/newsroom/news.aspx?id=d0be9be3-b4ef-46ae-bfe3-e2f5c10ac959

Case 37

Healthy Lifestyles Start at Home

CASE CONTRIBUTOR Scott D. Musch

Situation

Andrew, a lifestyle coach at a community Family YMCA, has started a meeting with a mother and her 10-year-old son to discuss the YMCA's new program, Healthy Family Home. Kristi, the program director at the Family YMCA, is also in attendance since Andrew is new with the organization and this is his first time personally consulting with members. After introductions, it is apparent to Andrew that the son is overweight, and may even be obese for his age, but he cannot make that determination definitively without weighing the child. The mother also appears overweight. The mother begins discussing her frustration with her son's weight as she feels helpless over the situation and is concerned that his weight will only get worse. Her son fidgets in his chair as his mother talks. They are obviously sensitive about the issue, and Andrew needs to be cautious with how he discusses the topic of obesity prevention and healthy living. In addition, although Kristi is sitting in the background quietly listening, Andrew knows she is monitoring his personal interactions with the family. Kristi places a high value on members feeling comfortable with her staff so that they will be encouraged to participate in the programs offered by the YMCA. Families such as this one need positive, ongoing support to make healthy living a reality in their lives, and Kristi wants the community YMCA to be a primary resource to them.

Instead of beginning the discussion with a series of questions about the family's eating habits and physical activities at home, which may be perceived as an interrogation, Andrew starts his discussion with the recognition of the many challenges families face. Families are busy and they confront many barriers to healthy lifestyles, including long work hours, overscheduled activities, unsafe neighborhoods, and poor eating choices. Andrew suggests that a solution to overcome these challenges is to make incremental changes toward incorporating healthy activities into family routines. The Healthy Family Home initiative is a program that can help families adopt and maintain healthy behaviors by taking small steps using the tools and resources developed by the YMCA. These tools revolve around The Pillars of a Healthy Family Home:[1]

- Eat Healthy
- Play Every Day
- Get Together
- Go Outside
- Sleep Well

Each pillar presents examples of objectives for a family to work toward together. They are realistic and achievable goals that recognize that the busiest of families can discover small ways to live healthier. Andrew recommends that the family set goals together each week and keep track of their performance in each of the pillars.

Background

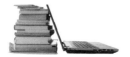

The YMCA (also referred to as the "Y") is a nonprofit community-based, cause-driven organization that promotes programs for youth development, healthy living, and social responsibility. The YMCA's "mission is to put Christian principles into practice through programs that build healthy spirit, mind and body for all."[2] The YMCA operates on the belief that a strong community can only be achieved by investing in our children, health, and neighbors. In the United States, the Y comprises the YMCA of the USA, a national resource office, and more than 2600 YMCAs with approximately 20,000 full-time staff and 500,000 volunteers in 10,000 communities across the country.[2] The Y engages 21 million men, women, and children—regardless of age, income, or background.[2]

During the past four decades, obesity rates have soared among all age groups, increasing more than fourfold among children ages 6 to 11, and today, nearly a third of children and adolescents are overweight or obese, representing more than 23 million kids and teenagers.[3] The prevalence of childhood obesity is a great public health concern as obesity tracks from childhood into adulthood, resulting in significant personal, social, and economic costs. A recent study projected that obesity will account for more than 16% of all healthcare expenditures by 2030.[4]

There are many public health initiatives and programs aimed at addressing this epidemic. The YMCA's Healthy Family Home initiative is centered on the understanding that healthy living begins at home. An objective of the initiative is to support families to sustain healthy lifestyles, as the relationship between a parent and child is a primary source for positive healthy behaviors. It can also serve as a motivator for adult parents to be healthier in their own lives to set an example for their children. Many families, however, need help and direction on how to build health into their lives. Through the program, the YMCA has made an effort to ensure that families are equipped with the tools and knowledge to create healthy environments. The YMCA recognizes that a one-size-fits-all strategy will not work for all families.

Next Steps

After the discussion, Andrew gives the mother and son a Healthy Family Home Starter Kit, which explains each of the five pillars and provides family goals examples. The family seems positive about the program and expresses interest in reading the material. Kristi appears happy with their reaction and smiles encouragingly at Andrew as they leave his office. Andrew hopes the family will take an active interest in adopting the self-directed program and will reach out to him for more information, tips, and activities along the way. He plans to recommend some fitness activities at the Y for the son, and perhaps even for the mother, during their next visit. Although Andrew is positive about the meeting, he realizes that the many barriers of everyday lives can present formidable obstacles to change.

He hopes to have the opportunity to continue his discussions with the son as well as support the family on its continuing journey toward making healthy living a top priority.

Discussion Questions

1. What are the goals of the YMCA's Healthy Family Home initiative? What might be some of the benefits and challenges of this type of public health program that concentrates on the family unit?

2. If you were Andrew, how might you have engaged the family to adopt and maintain healthy habits?

3. As Andrew's supervisor, how would you evaluate his communication approach with the family?

4. Should Andrew have asked if the family had access to regular primary health care?

5. What actions can public health professionals take to help facilitate changing unhealthy family behaviors?

References

[1] YMCA of the USA. (2010). *Build a Healthy Family Home*. Retrieved from the YMCA of the USA at http://www.ymca.net/healthy-family-home/

[2] YMCA of the USA. (2010). *Facts & Figures*. Retrieved from the YMCA of the USA at http://www.ymca.net/organizational-profile/

[3] Robert Wood Johnson Foundation. (2010). Retrieved from http://www.rwjf.org/childhoodobesity/challenge.jsp

[4] Wang, Y., Beydoun, M. A., Liang, L., Caballero, B., & Kumanyika, S. K. (2008, October). Will all Americans become overweight or obese? Estimating the progression and cost of the US obesity epidemic. *Obesity, 16*(10), 2323–2330.

Case 38

Transition Planning for Foster Youth with Special Health Care Needs

CASE CONTRIBUTOR Cynthia E. Harris

Situation

Dr. Louisa Smith, the medical director at the local child welfare agency, had received data indicating that only 50% of youth with special health care needs had received transition planning as they aged out of the system. Children or youth with special health care needs (CSHCN) are defined as "those children and youth who have or are at increased risk for a chronic physical, developmental, behavioral, or emotional condition and who also require health and related services of a type or amount beyond that required by children generally."[1] These foster children are wards of the state and are placed in protective services due to parental or caregiver neglect and/or abuse.

All children entering and exiting the child welfare system are required to have physical examinations. The child welfare system contracts with a local hospital to complete the entrance examinations. Dr. Smith is responsible for ensuring that children and youth in the system receive the medical and behavioral health services identified during entrance examinations. For children and youth with special health care needs, these services may include the need for having access to a medical home; receiving coordination to ensure their health, education, and child welfare needs are met; having adequate health insurance to cover all of their specialist and subspecialist referrals; and receiving transition planning prior to their aging out of the child welfare system. Follow-up for identified physical and psychological conditions is the responsibility of the assigned social worker and foster parent with whom the child or youth is placed. Social workers are either agency employees or employees of community-based child welfare agencies. Based on agency practice, Dr. Smith is not always made aware of whether or not follow-up care is received. This occurs due to the high volume of agency social work caseloads and poor communication with contracted private child welfare agencies.

Background

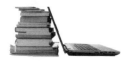

Youth with special health care needs and their families need help with transition planning. A transition plan is a written documentation by the time a child is 14 years old that includes what services need to be provided, who will provide them, and how they will be financed.[2] The plan addresses the transfer of medical care as well as the educational, recreational, and vocational opportunities that will facilitate a successful transition. Dr. Smith is not sure whether or not the youth overseen by her agency are receiving proper health transition planning. She is concerned that, as a member of the American Academy of Pediatrics (AAP), child welfare and educational transition planning regulations and policies differ from her trade organization. To illustrate, when youth transition from the child welfare system, they are required to have counseling concerning their transition beginning at age 16 with a focus on independent living. According to the Individuals with Disabilities Education Act, educational transition planning should begin at age 16 with focus on educational planning. Child welfare and education policies and regulations do not focus on the youth's health transition and begin later than recommended by the AAP and the Maternal and Child Health Bureau of the U.S. Health Resources and Services Administration. Dr. Smith believes that the agency should adopt the AAP's policy as it encompasses the health as well as the education and independent living needs of the youth.

Furthermore, as a result of these divergent regulations, policies, and laws, there is no coordination across these three systems—child welfare, health, and education. Due to the lack of coordination between systems, foster parents are often required to interact with personnel from several different agencies. Other than ensuring that youth with special health care needs are referred for medical and mental health services, social workers may not be aware if health or educational transition is occurring. Their focus is generally on transitioning youth as they age out of the foster care system. Once a youth has been placed in a foster home, Dr. Smith is often unaware of the physical and behavioral health referrals provided by internal and external social workers to foster parents for external healthcare providers. As a result, there is no centralized mechanism to determine whether or not transition planning is occurring or at what age it occurs.

In order to determine if transition planning was occurring across all systems involved in the child's life, Dr. Smith conducted a study with foster parents. Based on prior research in the field, she was aware that "youth in foster care transitioning out of the child welfare system are at risk of victimization, poverty, homelessness, early pregnancy, physical and mental health problems, poor access to health care, unemployment, and incarceration."[3] Dr. Smith's findings suggested that health transition planning was being conducted for only 50% of the youth. Therefore, she wanted to develop a plan to increase transition planning to a minimum of 85% to prevent some of the social and health issues experienced by so many youth as they age out of the system and to broaden the scope of transition planning beyond independent living. Dr. Smith is of the opinion that all systems can coordinate transition planning collaboratively. At the time of her research, Dr. Smith was not sure how many children and youth who entered the system had a special health care need, but she estimated it was likely between 31.0% and 50.3%.

Next Steps

Following up on her study, Dr. Smith has committed to develop a plan for the agency to address the need for transition planning for youth with special health care needs. Among the many factors necessary to evaluate in developing her plan, she recognizes that it will be critical to consider the various systems that interface with the youth and their foster parents.

Discussion Questions

1. What steps should Dr. Smith take to begin development of the plan to address the need for better transition planning across and within agencies?

2. Who are the key stakeholders who should be involved in the strategic planning process?

3. Who should take the leadership role in the planning process and why? How should a planning process incorporate the need to coordinate responsibility and accountability across different agencies, particularly if all the agencies have the same level of authority?

4. In light of the need to coordinate with internal and external stakeholders, what are some potential barriers that Dr. Smith will encounter?

5. In what ways can she manage through or overcome these barriers?

References

[1] McPherson, M., Arango, P., Fox, H., Lauver, C., McManus, M., Newacheck, P. W., . . . Strickland, B. (1998, July). A new definition of children with special health care needs. *Pediatrics, 102*(1), 137–139.

[2] Council on Children with Disabilities, American Academy of Pediatrics. (2005, November). Care coordination in the medical home: Integrating health and related systems of care for children with special health care needs. *Pediatrics, 116*(5), 1238–1244.

[3] Harris, C. E. (2009). *Determinates of health transition planning for foster youth with special health care needs in the District of Columbia.* (Doctoral dissertation).

Case 39

CASE CONTRIBUTOR Asal Mohamadi

Situation

The Florida Department of Health (DOH) has created a new division entitled the Department of Development and Sustainability (DDS). One of the responsibilities of the new department is to address rising trends in poor health across the state as they relate to the built environment. DDS would like to approach this mission at the municipal level by building community coalitions that provide for the capacity to address these health issues by working together to effect change. A coalition is an agreement among individuals or groups, during which they cooperate in joint action, each in their own self-interest, joining forces together for a common cause. DDS suggests that addressing health at the community level will eventually reverse some of these undesirable trends and promote a sustainable health profile for the state. To realize this goal DDS proposes a program called Healthy Communities, Healthy Citizens. This will consist of a conglomerate of smaller city level programs that address the needs of that particular city through coalitions consisting of members and organizations from the community.

Elizabeth Ruth was recently named the director of Healthy Communities, Healthy Citizens and has been charged with engineering and implementing the program. In order to obtain budget approval for the fund of Healthy Communities, Healthy Citizens, the program must first implement a successful pilot program.

Background

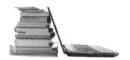

Tallahassee is the capital of Florida and has an approximate population of 180,000. Along with a multitude of state and city government agencies, Tallahassee hosts two major universities, State University and A&M University, one public and one private hospital, and a county health department. Elizabeth plans to implement a pilot program in Tallahassee called Citizens for a Healthy Tallahassee. If the pilot program proves successful, it will be implemented in cities and communities across the state.

Next Steps

Elizabeth would like to work with the City of Tallahassee to promote, among other things, physical activity, reduce vehicular dependency, and reduce alcohol and tobacco use. Elizabeth recognizes that Tallahassee is a heterogonous population with its citizenship having multiple cultures and interests. Identifying a representative list of stakeholders (individuals or organizations that have a stake in the mission of the program) proves imperative for successful implementation and to achieve the desired health outcomes. She also recognizes that to affect greater change, policies are needed that promote healthy behavior and address socioeconomic issues such as neighborhood concentrated poverty and neighborhood safety. It is important that the coalition be able to address the entire gambit of issues affecting health and the built environment.

Discussion Questions

1. Identify at least five health issues that may be related to the built environment. Explain how the built environment could possibly affect the identified health issue.

2. Identify at least 10 possible stakeholders (individuals or organizations that have a stake in the mission of the program) that could form a coalition.

3. Formulate a mission statement for the coalition that addresses identified health issues from Question 1 and accounts for stakeholders identified in Question 2.

Case 40   Medical Care Taking Flight

CASE CONTRIBUTOR **Margaret Ozan Rafferty**

Situation

As the plane leveled off, Mike Brooks reclined his seat and pulled out his notes and laptop. He had just spent three days in Turkey meeting with executives from International Kent Hospital ("Kent Hospital") and touring the medical facility's campus and was very impressed. As the vice president for Administration and Human Capital at Tastee International Beverage, Mike was responsible for the benefits of the company's 25,000 worldwide employees and their families. As a self-insured employer, Tastee International Beverage manages its own health insurance benefits for employees and their dependents. Over the past six years, the organization had seen a fourfold increase in their medical insurance costs and Mike was charged with creating a cost reduction plan to be implemented in the upcoming fiscal year.

Earlier in the year, Mike had attended a conference on emerging trends in medical care options. At the conference, he participated in a breakout session on a growing trend called medical tourism. He learned that while it sounded like a new term, "medical tourism" or traveling for care, had centuries of history starting in ancient times when people had sought out the healing waters of therapeutic spas. In the last century, wealthy individuals traveled to the United States for specialty care and to countries in South America for cosmetic surgery. However, more recently, hospitals overseas are becoming viable options for patients seeking affordable quality health care.

One of the presenters at the breakout session was from a hospital in Thailand. He shared that over the past few years his organization provided care for over 400,000 international patients. Nearly all the physicians in the health system spoke English and over 200 were U.S. board certified. Another presenter, a representative from Turkey, boasted that his country had the highest number of Joint Commission International (JCI) accredited hospitals. He highlighted Turkey's cost-effective options for orthopedic, fertility, and eye surgeries. During the question and answer session, the audience asked the panelists about quality and costs, and they heard many examples of positive outcomes and significant cost savings. In addition, the presenters from the various countries highlighted their hospitals' amenities and stressed that they provided a very high level of customer service for their international patients.

Upon returning home from the conference, Mike's interest in medical tourism was piqued. He immersed himself in learning more about the options for healthcare procedures outside the United States. He learned that many hospitals overseas have made attracting international patients a key strategic initiative. They provide patients with high-tech equipment, comparable to that found in the United States, coupled with immaculate facilities at lower costs. In addition to the potential cost savings, patients often seek care in another country to avoid long wait times, obtain a service not covered by their health insurance plans, or have a procedure not offered in their own country.

Mike was surprised to learn that many foreign medical facilities have affiliations with U.S. healthcare systems such as the Johns Hopkins Health System and the Cleveland Clinic. He also learned that medical tourism facilitators often serve as intermediaries between patients and hospitals, and they provide extensive details on these service providers. Facilitators have typically visited the hospitals and have screened the facilities for quality and service. Cost for care in these international facilities is typically packaged together by these facilitators and include airfare, hotel for additional recovery, and often accommodations for a family member. Mike also read that many of these facilitators note on their websites that they would do everything possible to address an adverse outcome if the patient was still in the facility, and several had relationships with providers in the United States for coordinating any follow-up care.

Mike thought this all sounded too good to be true. Quality health care at lower prices was exactly what he wanted for his employees and their families. He decided to explore medical tourism providers in greater detail. He called several of the medical tourism facilitators he met at the conference. They provided him with additional resources and encouraged him to personally visit a medical tourism provider. Mike got a chuckle out of the thought of going to his boss and asking to take a trip overseas as part of the organization's cost reduction initiatives. However, once he presented the background information and outlined the potential cost savings associated with a medical tourism option, Mike's boss approved the expenditure and Mike booked a trip to Turkey to visit Kent Hospital.

Background

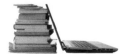

After a very pleasant direct flight to Turkey on Turkish Airlines, Mike was met at the airport by Yasemin, a patient representative of Kent Hospital. Yasemin explained that she wanted Mike to experience Kent Hospital like an international patient, without going through an actual procedure, of course. As they drove to the hospital, Yasemin shared that Kent Hospital was constructed in 2004 and was built according to the American Institute of Architect guidelines and JCI standards. Consultants from the Mayo Clinic were enlisted to launch the hospital's initial medical guidelines and administrative protocols. Less than two years after opening, the hospital received its initial JCI accreditation and has continued to receive ongoing accreditation thereafter. The hospital has 160 beds and a medical staff of over 90. Most of the medical staff and a large portion of the nurses are fluent in English and the majority of the department heads received training in the United Kingdom or the United States.

As they pulled up to the hospital, Mike was very impressed. The grounds were immaculate and they were greeted with a cheery "Welcome to Kent" by a volunteer at the entrance. The lobby boasted a grand piano with light music played by a gentleman in a tuxedo. Moving through the hospital, Mike noticed that everyone he met made eye contact and said hello. Yasemin took him to "his room," where Mike could not believe the modern furnishing and breathtaking panoramic views from the large windows. After less than a minute, a nurse knocked on the door, came in, introduced herself, and provided Mike with a detailed orientation to the unit and completed his admission assessment.

After the nurse showed Mike the bedside computer system and electronic medical record, Yasemin took Mike on a tour of the hospital. He saw modern equipment and professional staff in every department. Members of the medical and nursing staff were eager to talk about their patient outcomes, quality, and their high levels of patient satisfaction. Returning to the room, a young woman from food service came in to take his order for dinner from a menu with a variety of options. Mike stayed the night in the hospital room and was pleasantly surprised at the responsiveness of the nursing staff and how well he slept.

The following day, Mike spent the morning with representatives of the international patient department and after a delicious lunch in the hospital's restaurant, he met with senior leadership. He was very impressed with the organization's transparency and willingness to share their outcomes and quality data, which they benchmark against Turkish and international standards. Mike learned that the hospital created packages for most procedures. These packages consisted of travel, hospital, surgical, physician, and pre- and postoperative hotel lodging costs. Accommodations for a spouse or significant other were also included. Mike was intrigued to learn that the price for an all-inclusive package for coronary bypass at Kent Hospital was approximately $15,000. Mike knew costs for the same procedure in U.S. major cities were well over $60,000. A review of the hospital's prices for other procedures such as hip and knee replacements showed similar potential savings.

After another night in the hospital, Mike spent his last full day in Turkey touring the local sites and learning more about Turkey's history. The hospital arranged for Mike to spend his last night in town at a local hotel where patients typically recover after their inpatient stay. Again, Mike was impressed with the service and hospitality at the hotel.

Next Steps

The seat-belt light switched off and the Turkish Airline flight attendant approached Mike to take his beverage order. As he sipped his Tastee Cola, Mike knew he had some major decisions to make on the flight home. Would adding a medical tourism option for his employees make sense?

Discussion Questions

1. Explain the possible benefits of adding medical tourism to the organization's medical plan.

2. Describe the risks involved in adding a medical tourism option. Consider the perspective from the viewpoint of a self-insured employer and as an employer with stewardship and responsibility for its employees.

3. As a manager of a health plan benefit design, what should Mike consider as he decides whether to implement a medical tourism option?

4. Describe how healthcare reform may affect the growth of medical tourism.

5. What factors would a health insurance company need to consider in implementing a medical tourism option that a self-insured company might not need to consider?

Case 41   Rural Health Care in Central Michigan

CASE CONTRIBUTOR **Jessica Gardon Rose**

Situation

The University of Wisconsin Population Health Institute, in collaboration with the Robert Wood Johnson Foundation, released the first nationwide *County Health Rankings Report* in February 2010.[1] The rankings report is a collection of 50 state reports comparing the health rankings of counties within each state. This study, which is to be continued for at least two more years, provides a barometer of overall health and the factors that influence health, including clinical care, health behaviors, socioeconomic factors, and the physical environment. According to the institute's researchers, the report "shows us that where we live matters to our health. The health of a community depends on many different factors— ranging from individual health behaviors, education and jobs, to quality of health care, to the environment."[2]

The county health rankings are a key component of the Mobilizing Action Toward Community Health (MATCH) project.[3] MATCH helps state and local health departments mobilize local community leaders and residents to invest in developing action plans for addressing barriers to health and helping people lead healthier lifestyles.

In central Michigan, Mary Kushion, health officer for the Central Michigan District Health Department (CMDHD), was very concerned with the *County Health Rankings Report*, since the study revealed that the six counties within the health department's district were in critical need of healthcare improvement (see Figure 41–1).[4] On average, the health rankings of counties within the CMDHD area were worse than 79% of the Michigan counties outside of the district, with Clare County in central Michigan ranked as the unhealthiest in the state.

In response to the report, the CMDHD embarked upon an effort to improve the overall health of the more than 187,000 individuals within the geographical range of its healthcare operations. CMDHD initiated the aptly named Together We Can (TWC) community campaign, calling for stakeholders to collaboratively embark on a new community-wide process to improve the health and quality of life of residents in their communities.[5] In partnership with Central Michigan University (CMU), CMDHD, and community health centers in the six-county district, the TWC Health Improvement Council is working to create a districtwide health improvement plan through the pooling of community health assessments and health improvement plans. This districtwide health plan is expected to prioritize key health issues, establish action plans for addressing barriers to health, and develop strategies for helping residents in the six-county district lead healthier lifestyles.

Figure 41–1 Michigan Health Outcomes Map

Central Michigan County Health Rankings (outlined in **White**)

82 – Clare
77 – Gladwin
72 – Arenac
70 – Roscommon
45 – Osceola
42 – Isabella

Source: *County Health Rankings by Local Health Department* (February 2010).[6]

Background

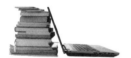

The mission of the CMDHD is to "promote health & physical well-being by providing preventative health care, education, & environmental safety to all members of the community."[7] Despite the economic downturn, Health Officer Mary Kushion has ensured that CMDHD continues to provide quality healthcare services to clients in its six-county district. The health department team consists of dedicated registered nurses, nurse practitioners, dentists, dietitian, social workers, environmental sanitarians, and health educators working with community and clinical student volunteers to provide a wide variety of personal health, dental, family planning, environmental health, health promotion, and emergency preparedness services.

Access to health care for vulnerable populations remains challenging due to the current economic depression of the state. The six-county district is plagued by a high incidence of cardiovascular disease, cancer, and diabetes. Top health factor issues include obesity, binge drinking, and tobacco use. The *County Health Rankings Report* revealed problems of unemployment (6–12% throughout central Michigan), lack of healthcare coverage (11–17%), and limited schooling, with only approximately 12% pursuing a bachelor's degree or higher (as compared to 83% in Michigan as a whole).[4,8]

Nearly one in five central Michigan residents (21%) was identified to be of low income in 2009, as compared to 16% of total Michigan residents and 14% of the nation as a whole.[8] In the same year, approximately 32% of central Michigan county children under age 18 were living in poverty, as compared to 22% of children in Michigan and 20% of children in the United States.

Many low-income families have trouble accessing healthcare services due to lack of health insurance to cover primary healthcare needs. In turn, local health providers experience financial difficulties and often leave to practice medicine elsewhere. This is what has been happening in central Michigan's rural counties and small communities, which are federally designated as Primary Care Professional Shortage Areas, Dental Care Health Professional Shortage Areas, Mental Health Professional Shortage Areas, and Medically Underserved Areas/Populations.[9,10]

Faced with high rates of poverty, an aging population, a vulnerable local economy, and substantial healthcare access barriers, Health Officer Mary Kushion has asked for help from the TWC team. She has asked for TWC to establish objectives and identify the target resident stakeholders of focus. In addition, TWC has been charged with identifying those stakeholders who need to come to the table to influence change for implementing action plans to improve health outcomes in central Michigan. CMDHD also needs concrete timelines and identification of outcome measures for monitoring how the TWC campaign is progressing.

Next Steps

The campaign is a large undertaking and TWC has many management challenges to overcome. Where does TWC start? What groups or individuals should be involved in order to have a truly representative community organization? How can TWC facilitate consistency with discussions and planning development when volunteers need to travel significant distances to get to meetings? How can health outcome statistical reports be compiled for the lay community to easily interpret and understand? How can TWC engage a diverse group of stakeholders? How can the group maintain momentum and ensure goal-oriented progress on its work?

TWC needs to apply team leadership techniques and community-based participatory research processes for developing a long-term collaborative research and action agenda. To help build the TWC infrastructure and skills needed to move forward with the campaign, Health Officer Mary Kushion has asked for support from CMU.

The early stages of the TWC project have been supported by in-kind donations and volunteer efforts by stakeholders. Their efforts have resulted in a preliminary examination of conditions in the central Michigan county district. However, the development of an organized research and action agenda requires a more in-depth understanding of local factors including residents' and providers' perceptions of community needs and community readiness. This can be readily accomplished through the implementation of comprehensive community assessments and community-action practices associated with community-based participatory research.[11]

Having trained leaders and the key resources required to implement and evaluate program interventions will be crucial to successfully improve the health outcomes of central Michigan residents. The need to have additional trained leaders to coordinate group meetings, facilitate community-based focus groups, manage collected data, and develop action plans is strongly evident. Unfortunately, few members of the otherwise excellent staff of the CMDHD are trained in conducting community health assessment activities. The CMDHD partnership with CMU will result in the application of team leadership training and community-based research mechanisms needed for ramping up focused community team performance.

In the few months since launching the TWC initiative, team leadership recognized the need for audio and video telecommunication equipment in order to have members participate from remote locations when they were unable to participate in person. A virtual team room supported on a web-based platform allows for effective information exchange and collaboration through the sharing of documents, project management timetables, resources, and an up-to-date list of active team members.[12] To support development of the virtual team platform, CMU is assisting TWC with grant procurement, technical support, and educational resources to enhance team building and open information exchange.

The establishment of a centralized data warehouse and information portal for community stakeholders and researchers is also planned. The portal, to be maintained by CMDHD, will allow one-stop accessing of federal and state data, as well as local county health outcomes data. This portal will be important for enabling county stakeholders to not only monitor the outcomes of their health improvement plan initiatives, but also to review the best practices established by neighboring communities. CMU resources will be able to assist in supporting information exchange and development of this portal for facilitating improved health outcomes in central Michigan.

The strategy plan has been established for TWC. The team waits to see over the next several years the outcomes of the TWC campaign. Hopefully, as a result of well-organized team collaboration and effective project management, victory will be realized.

Discussion Questions

1. How would you prioritize the issues that affect health and health outcomes in rural counties and small communities?

2. What issues can the TWC team tackle locally versus those that require assistance from more influential stakeholders at the state and federal level?

3. How can the goals of various interest groups be aligned to buy into the TWC campaign?

4. Given the various factors affecting community health outcomes, what stakeholders should be included in the TWC Health Improvement Council and its community health planning workgroup subcommittees?

5. What are some of the challenges faced by the health department in implementing TWC?

6. There are several challenges that the TWC team may face when operating in a virtual environment. What strategies will help TWC with planning, team communication, and decision making?

7. What strategies should the TWC team employ to improve health outcomes in communities where healthy lifestyles and improving health are not seen as priorities to many of the residents?

8. Given that funding is limited to support public health programs, are there policies and laws that could be implemented to improve a community's health infrastructure and promote healthier lifestyles?

References

[1] University of Wisconsin Population Health Institute. (2010). *County health rankings—About this project*. Retrieved from University of Wisconsin's Population Health Institute County Health Rankings at http://www.countyhealthrankings.org/about-project

[2] University of Wisconsin Population Health Institute. (n.d.). *MATCH activities*. Retrieved from the University of Wisconsin's Population Health Institute County Health Rankings at http://uwphi .pophealth.wisc.edu/pha/match/activities.htm

[3] University of Wisconsin Population Health Institute. (n.d.). *Mobilizing action toward community health (MATCH): Population health metrics, solid partnerships, and real incentives*. Retrieved from the University of Wisconsin's Population Health Institute County Health Rankings at http://uwphi.pophealth.wisc.edu/pha/match.htm

[4] University of Wisconsin Population Health Institute. (2010, February). *County health rankings—Mobilizing action toward community health: 2010 Michigan*. Retrieved from the University of Wisconsin's Population Health Institute County Health Rankings at http://www .countyhealthrankings.org/Michigan

[5] Central Michigan District Health Department. (2010). *A healthy community—Together We Can! County health rankings information for the Central Michigan District Health Department counties Arenac, Clare, Gladwin, Isabella, Osceola and Roscommon*. Retrieved from http://www.cmdhd.org

[6] Michigan Department of Community Health. (2010, February). *County health rankings by local health department*.Retrieved from http://www.michigan.gov/documents/mdch/County_Health_ Outcome_Rank_LHD_Final_311627_7.pdf

[7] Central Michigan District Health Department. (2010, April). Agency brochure. Retrieved from http://www.cmdhd.org/contact/aboutus

[8] United States Census Bureau. (2009). Small area income and poverty estimates—State and county estimates for 2009. Retrieved from http://www.census.gov/did/www/saipe/data/statecounty/ data/2009.html

[9] Health Resources and Services Administration. (2010, May). *Shortage designation: HPSAs, MUAs & MUPs*. Retrieved from the United States Department of Health and Human Services at http://bhpr.hrsa.gov/shortage

[10] State of Michigan. (2001, April). *Urban/Rural designation for Michigan counties*. Retrieved from the State of Michigan at http://www.michigan.gov/documents/urban_rural_50265_7.pdf

[11] Eng, E., & Blanchard, L. (2007). Action-oriented community diagnosis: A health education tool. *International Quarterly of Community Health Education, 26*(2), 141–158.

[12] Prevou, M., Veitch, R. H., & Sullivan, R. F. (2009). *Teams of leaders: Raising the level of collaborative leader-team performance*. Paper presented at the Interservice/Industry Training, Simulation, and Education Conference. Abstract retrieved from http://www.teamsofleaders.org/Resources.html

Case 42 | Smoking Cessation Program Implementation

CASE CONTRIBUTOR **James Allen Johnson, III**

Situation

Dr. Whitten is the director of a community health clinic in Lake Sophia, Florida. Lake Sophia is a small town with approximately 2,000 residence located in a rural area of central Florida. The town of Lake Sophia is located in one of the poorest areas in the state. The health of the population of Lake Sophia reflects its socioeconomic status (SES) in that not only does it have some of the lowest SES indicators (income, education, and occupation) in Florida, but its population has some of the worst health as well.

Dr. Whitten was concerned about a report recently released by the State Department of Health on tobacco use. The report indicated that 32% of the population in Lake Sophia used tobacco. This statistic was not only well above the national average of approximately 20%, but was the highest in the state. In response to this revelation about the significance of the problem of tobacco use in Lake Sophia, Dr. Whitten decided to implement a smoking cessation program at the health clinic.

To develop, implement, and eventually manage the program, Dr. Whitten hired Ali Jones, a recent college graduate who majored in Public Health. Remembering her public health education, Ali concluded that to ensure success she must use an evidence-based approach. She decided to refer to recent literature written about smoking cessation as well as the Centers for Disease Control and Prevention (CDC) and the World Health Organization (WHO) websites.

Background

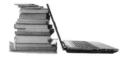

Ali concluded the consensus was that tobacco dependence showed many features of a chronic disease and that only a minority of tobacco users achieves successful cessation while the majority continues to use tobacco long-term, typically cycling through multiple periods of relapse and remission. Further inquiry revealed that only about 5% of smokers who quit smoking maintained abstinence for 3 to 12 months.[1] It is suggested by the American Cancer Society that one of the reasons for the low success rate may be attributed to the fact that most individuals who try to quit do not use effective treatments.[2] In 2000, the U.S. Public Health Service published and in 2008 updated *Guidelines for Treating Tobacco Use and Dependence*, which includes both recommended treatment strategies for clinicians and implementation stages for administrators.

Next Steps

Ali adopted the recommended treatment strategies from the *Guidelines for Treating Tobacco Use and Dependence* and had all the clinicians and practitioners at the health clinic properly trained. The program seemed to be going well but Ali knew there was room for improvement. She noticed that on breaks, some of the employees of the clinic would sit on benches near the front entrance and smoke cigarettes. This was a designated smoking area and next to the benches ashtrays were provided. Ali realized that to further the success of the smoking cessation program she must employ a systemic approach. To help in the formulation of ideas for a systems intervention approach, Ali called a meeting that included clinicians, practitioners, and administrators.

Discussion Questions

1. Discuss some possible opportunities and concerns Ali may want to introduce at the meeting.

2. What are some possible opportunities and concerns the other participants at the meeting (clinicians, practitioners, and administrators) may have?

3. Should Ali address the issue of employees smoking outside in front of the building? Why or why not? If so, what changes should she recommend and how should they be implemented?

References

[1] Centers for Disease Control and Prevention. (2006). *A practical guide to working with health-care systems on tobacco-use treatment*. Retrieved from http://www.cdc.gov/tobacco/quit_smoking/ cessation/practical_guide/pdfs/practical_guide.pdf

[2] American Cancer Society. (2003). *Cancer facts and figures, 2003*. Atlanta, GA: American Cancer Society.

Case 43

CASE CONTRIBUTOR James A. Johnson

Situation

Dr. Hartman, the only cardiologist in the small town of Sparton, IL, has an office with a staff of three in the cardiology department of the local community hospital.[1] He has numerous patients but is not certified to perform commonly recommended cardiac catheterizations. Therefore, he must refer his patients to other practices in Belleville, which is 30 miles away. Dr. Hartman refers most of his patients to a large five-physician practice, Belleville Cardiology; in return, Belleville Cardiology takes his calls whenever he is out of town or on a vacation.

Dr. Hartman recently began doing so much work with Belleville Cardiology's physicians that they decided to form a legal merger in which Dr. Hartman would be considered a partner of their group but would continue to operate his office. Because he was the only cardiologist in his town, this arrangement ensured Belleville Cardiology the opportunity to serve almost all the heart patients from that county. The physicians of Belleville Cardiology would also see patients one day per week in Sparton so that Dr. Hartman could increase his volume of patients.

After several meetings, a quick merger was conducted in which the six physicians became partners. The contract specified only some items. Details such as billing, patient charts, and records would be worked out later. The office staffs would remain the same at both offices, all six physicians would be salaried, and the practice would comprise the large Belleville office and the small hospital-based office in Sparton.

In the first month, several unanticipated problems presented themselves to the newly merged practice. Because the offices were more than 30 miles apart, planning and organizational meetings were difficult to schedule, but many decisions needed to be made. Changes in letterhead stationery, billing procedures, and patient information were made by Dr. Youngblood, president and founder of Belleville Cardiology, and his staff. Dr. Hartman's staff felt alienated because all these decisions were made without their input.

In addition, because of the distance between the offices, the office staffs had not met each other. They spoke only on the phone as needed to answer questions, exchange patient information, and make appointments. Both staffs also had loyalties to the particular physicians who had hired them. When Dr. Hartman called Belleville Cardiology's office manager with instructions, the manager never knew if Drs. Youngblood and Hartman had previously discussed the issue. She was not used to following instructions from someone new whom she had never met. Dr. Hartman's nurses had the same problems with Belleville Cardiology's doctors.

Moreover, the office staff was not familiar with the preferences of the physicians from the other office. For example, one physician might routinely check a treadmill patient's blood pressure 2 minutes into the exercise while another would check after 5 minutes. This difference caused some confusion, especially when Dr. Youngblood or his two partners worked at Dr. Hartman's office because they never had worked with his staff.

When his first paycheck arrived Dr. Hartman was dissatisfied because of the deductions of money owed to Belleville Cardiology for services performed by their physicians on his patients while he was on vacation. These services had been billed by his office. Dr. Hartman had agreed on the formula to be used to calculate his pay, but he had not anticipated the extent of the services the other physicians had performed. He was accustomed to taking home all the profits from his office rather than being paid a check for the same amount each month.

Discussion Questions

1. What are the most pressing issues of this situation?

2. What considerations should have been made for the post-merger integration of the staffs and office practices?

3. Who should take charge of the situation in the offices?

4. List some recommendations for improvements that should be made.

Reference

[1] Kilpatrick, A. O., & Johnson, J. A. (1999). *Human resources and organizational behavior: Cases in health services management*. Chicago, IL: Health Administration Press.

Case 44

CASE CONTRIBUTOR **James A. Johnson**

Situation

Figure 44–1 shows the organizational design for Lake Oswego Retirement Community, a continuing care retirement community (CCRC).[1] Created with input from the board of trustees, the executive director, and administrators, it represents a sincere and wrenching effort to enhance performance and match the design with the expanding organization's mission and strategies. The design maximizes individual talents and abilities through the positioning of services and linkage of responsibilities. The executive director, however, states that the intent of the design has been to protect areas of authority from other powerful individuals and to require coordination among designed services.

Figure 44–1 Organizational Design for Lake Oswego Retirement Community

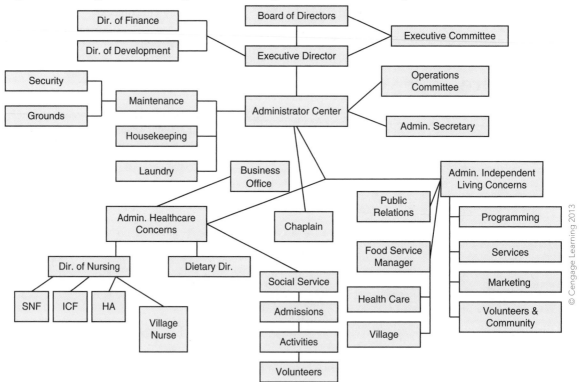

© Cengage Learning 2013

Background

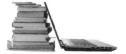

A CCRC is a particular type of retirement community that offers several levels of health care in one location. It includes a combination of independent living units (ILU) or assisted living facilities (ALF), and healthcare units (HCU) for skilled nursing and rehabilitation (both short- and long-term). For client purposes, a CCRC supplies retirement housing in a community setting linked to guaranteed health care in the HCU at a time when mental or physical abilities fail. The benefit to the organization is a dedicated population for the HCU. The HCU presence on campus is vital enough that retirement centers without a nursing care component have difficulties being marketed.

This vertical integration results in a nursing home next to a hotel or, more exactly, apartments. The continuum flows from the ILU to ALF to HCU. The units share common services (e.g., dietary, nursing, environmental, social, marketing) with distinctive orientations determined by unit population. For example, the dietary department, located in the HCU, prepares meals for all CCRC residents. State inspection surveys examine all services rendered in the nursing care facility. They require the dietary department to adhere to any special diets (e.g., low salt, diabetic, low cholesterol), serve warm meals, and provide assistance in eating when necessary. The same food is served to the ILU and ALF residents. They eat in a separate dining area with a cafeteria-restaurant atmosphere. The control at the ILU and ALF is not state inspection but the satisfaction of the clients. This population decides its own food preferences from what is available, and the dietary department decides whether it is good for them or not.

Another essential difference between the populations is the living arrangements. ILU and ALF residents live in apartments or cottages, pay monthly fees similar to rent, and may leave of their own volition at any time. In contrast, HCU residents are admitted only by order of a physician and are assigned to a licensed or certified bed in a room that is usually double occupancy. Payment may be through government reimbursement or commercial/private pay. If a patient wants to leave the HCU, an opening must first be found at another facility.

Next Steps

Lake Oswego Retirement Community, represented by the organizational chart, consists of a 100-bed HCU established 15 years ago as a nursing home. Within the last five years, 60 ILUs/ALFs, including both rooms and cottages, have been added. Currently, Lake Oswego Retirement Community is fully occupied and expanding with an additional 80 ILUs/ALFs, adult day care services, and a health clinic. The number of CCRCs has been increasing in the state, and management is concerned about the low occupancy rates of other facilities even though they do not compete in the same geographic area.

Discussion Questions

1. What are the problems with the design shown in the existing organization chart?

2. Suggest an organizational design appropriate for this organization. Draw a chart delineating duties and showing the reporting structure of the design.

3. Why will a different model work better?

Reference

[1] Kilpatrick, A. O., & Johnson, J. A. (1999). *Human resources and organizational behavior: Cases in health services management.* Chicago, IL: Health Administration Press.

Case 45

CASE CONTRIBUTOR **Adam Miller**

Situation

It had been a busy day for Lance, and he was certain that this was just a harbinger of things to come. As the youngest group product director in the company for one of the most anticipated anti-infective pharmaceutical medicines coming to market, the pressure was building to ensure a successful product launch. A swift uptake in the primary care and specialty provider regimen, both in the hospital and provider office settings, was an expected and financially necessary end goal. Recently promoted to his new position, Lance was responsible for all aspects of a product lifecycle, including coordinating the various teams required to ensure a successful launch. This role was one of the most difficult and precarious responsibilities in any pharmaceutical company. Matrix Pharmaceuticals ("Matrix"), like many others in the industry, was experiencing a drying of its product pipeline and had been losing market share to generic competition of its expiring patents. This new anti-infective was going to ensure the company was on a solid financial footing for years to come, and failure could mean a swift dissolution of the company to a rival buyout.

As he hurried from one tense meeting to the next, questions concerning needs, resources, and outcomes came at a rapid pace. The answers were complex, difficult, and almost as ambiguous as the marketplace the company was hoping to successfully enter under Lance's leadership. As a 15-year employee of Matrix, the fourth largest pharmaceutical company in North America, Lance had risen quickly within the commercial side of the corporate organization. This was due in part to his deep knowledge of both the science and the marketplace, but more due to his ability to quickly "take a pulse" on those he interacted with, and make appropriate decisions regardless of individual differences. While his MBA and MPH gave him the credentials to advance, his soft skills were what his colleagues attributed to his rapid and sustained organizational success. Indeed, as his exposure to senior management increased, he seemed destined to rise even further in the company, and a Matrix senior leadership vice president position seemed to be the next logical advance for Lance's career.

Today, however, the corporate ladder seemed to have run out of rungs for Lance. As he headed back to his office for a quick briefing on a recent anti-infective managed care payor landscape analysis, he had time to reflect on the project at hand. Problems seemed to be standard operating procedure for this product launch. The company's internal landscape had been significantly altered within days of Lance's promotion. The division leadership had been shaken up, resulting in changes in critical points of contact with which Lance had no or very little relationship. Additionally, the commercial business unit, along with group product directors including Lance, was now informed that the company would take a very conservative approach to sales and marketing activities and budget. However, the sales forecast for product sales was still being increased by at least 5% due to deteriorating currency values abroad. Lance had planned to leverage his global counterparts as part of a transnational advisory board, as the launch of the anti-infective was anticipated in the Europe and Asian markets. It was now apparent that the European Medicines Agency was not going to recommend approval of the agent, and his counterparts now had little time to work with Lance on the current project. Finally, the company had anticipated a new class designation for the novel anti-infective, which would have ensured coverage within Medicare Part D programs, a major share of Lance's anticipated revenue. Unfortunately, the WHO International Working Group for Drug Statistics Methodology had declined to issue a new Anatomical Therapeutic Chemical (ATC) classification system code. An ATC is a classification system in which the active substances are divided into different groups according to the organ or system on which they act and their therapeutic, pharmacological, and chemical properties. It was anticipated that this could have a major impact on how health insurance plans recognized and reimbursed the anti-infective for coverage and novel use.

Next Steps

These issues were not anticipated when Lance began the project. Using his previous launch modeling projections was useless. Lance realized he would need to adapt when it came to product launches in this new environment. He was deeply concerned about this complex and unpredictable environment. This represented a "new normal" environment in which the pharmaceutical industry was operating. As he tried to refocus on the landscape analysis, he put down the report and picked up the phone to call his mentor. He was certain his mentor would know how to handle this situation. Lance had the knowledge, skills, and ability to navigate through market changes, but he needed some reassurance that his instincts were correct. As the phone rang on the other end, Lance scribbled down some questions to which he needed quick answers.

Discussion Questions

1. What are the core issues that Lance must address to successfully launch the anti-infective? How should Lance prioritize these issues?

2. Lance seems very frustrated by the recent personnel and policy changes, and how they are affecting his launch planning. Should he have anticipated any of these problems? How should Lance have contingency planned?

3. What does Lance mean when he refers to the "new normal"? What are some steps he can take to successfully operate within this environment moving forward?

4. What organizational trends and decisions are impacting Lance? How could he plan to successfully navigate internally to achieve success?

5. How has the pharmaceutical industry changed over the past decade? How will today's executives and managers successfully navigate this change?

Group Exercise

In small groups (4–5 participants), simulate the following scenario:

As a member of the product launch advisory committee to Lance, each of you has been called by Lance to prepare him for a Monday morning meeting of the Matrix senior leadership to discuss the status of the product launch. Senior leadership has made it clear that they are concerned with recent developments and want to ensure that the project is on track and will be successfully executed. They are familiar with the external challenges that have been imposed on the product launch, and have requested a formal presentation of the current situation and an action plan for a remediation strategy. It is now Friday morning and you must work as a group to prepare Lance for this presentation. Design a presentation that takes the request into account. You will present your draft to Lance on Friday afternoon. Consider all variables, both that Lance will present to senior leadership and those that Lance should be aware of when presenting to senior leadership. The presentation must include a recommendation for an outcome action plan for each variable identified.

Case 46

CASE CONTRIBUTOR **John Brady**

Situation

Marianjoy Rehabilitation Hospital (Marianjoy) is an inpatient rehabilitation facility located in the western suburbs of Chicago. In fiscal year 2009, leadership at the facility noticed overall patient satisfaction had plateaued, placing the hospital at the 46th percentile as measured by Press Ganey. One area of particular concern to the leadership of Marianjoy was satisfaction with discharge planning and processes relating to the transitions between levels of care as it was lagging behind the overall hospital score (i.e., overall satisfaction for discharge questions was at the 39th percentile).

Background

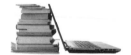

Marianjoy is a 108-bed inpatient rehabilitation facility, which also operates a 20-bed skilled nursing facility and outpatient rehabilitation services on its campus. The hospital is a member of the Wheaton Franciscan Health Care system (WFHC) based primarily in Wisconsin and Iowa, so it does not receive direct referrals from other WFHC facilities. Instead, Marianjoy relies on referral relationships from acute care hospitals located in the nearby area (i.e., within a roughly 15 mile radius). As a result, in order to meet the needs of its referral sources it is imperative for patients at Marianjoy to transition across the continuum of post-acute care services seamlessly while avoiding unnecessary readmissions to the acute care setting.

Approach to Challenge

To address the suboptimal satisfaction scores, a multidisciplinary team of leaders and associates was convened to collaborate on a service excellence strategy. Leaders from nursing, therapy, admissions, patient financial services, and outpatient services were included in this effort. The group was tasked with identifying a solution to the poor scores related to discharge planning and the transitions between levels of care. Each month the CEO of Marianjoy would be provided with an update on the group's progress and asked to provide any insight or input into the process.

As the Marianjoy Service Excellence team began investigating the issue, specific attention was paid to understanding the voice of the patients and their family/caregivers, as well as the application of quality principles and performance improvement based on data-driven evidence (e.g., clinical outcomes, patient perceptions of care). From these assessments, the team developed an enterprisewide strategy for service excellence that would extend across the continuum of post-acute care services offered through Marianjoy. The goal was to design a program to both improve the patient experience and bolster patient and family member understanding of what to expect during the inpatient rehabilitation stay and beyond. This strategy was called the "The Inpatient Journey Along the Rehabilitation Road to Discharge™" (Figure 46–1).

Figure 46–1 The Inpatient Journey Along the Rehabilitation Road to Discharge™

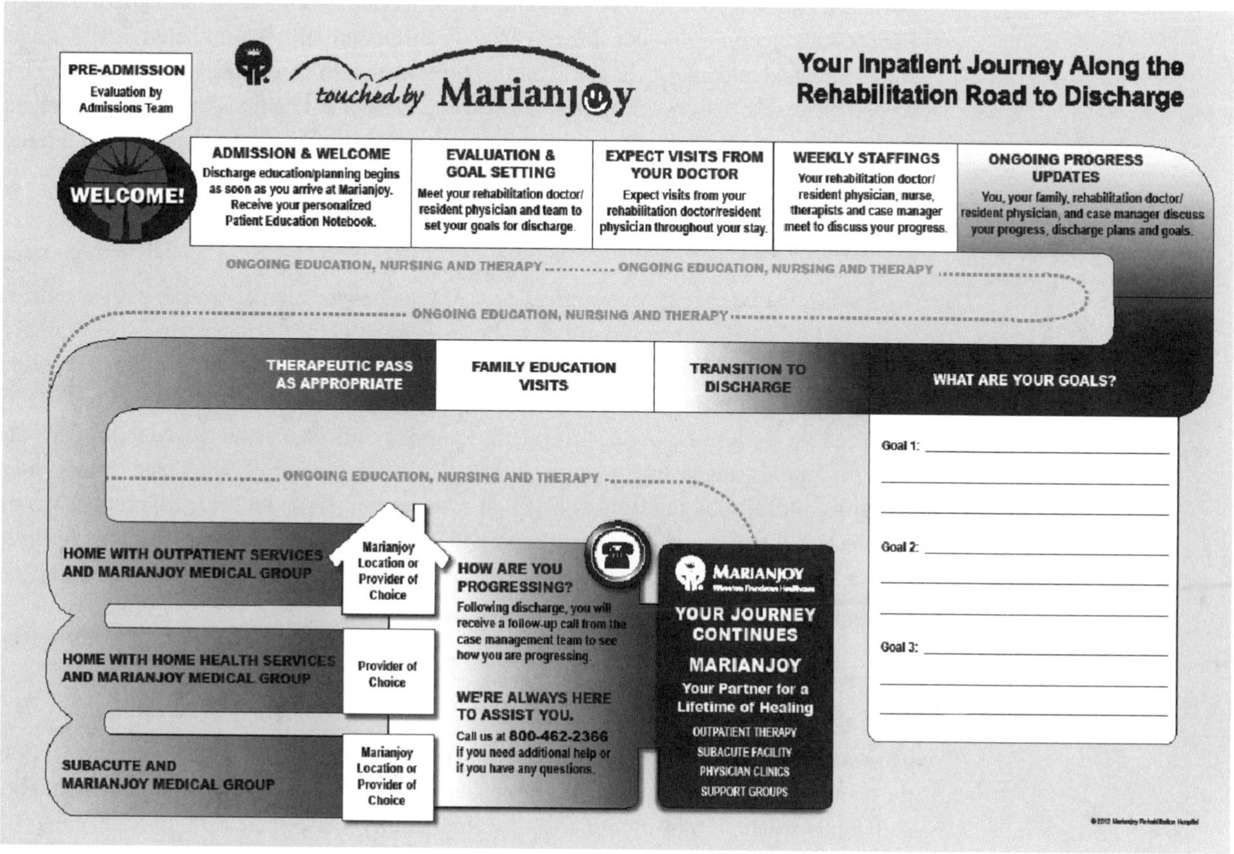

Reprinted with permission from Marianjoy.

Through this strategy, associates at Marianjoy are able to conceptualize and explain what the patients' experiences will be during their stay, and how they will continue their rehabilitation following discharge. Nursing, therapy, and medical staff were all educated and trained on how to reference the "Journey," and to remind patients their discharge planning and goal setting begins on the first day of their admission. Rehabilitation requires hard work on the part of the patient, and the "Journey" concept offers an understanding of what the payoff for that work will be. Further, it demonstrates to patients how they will move between the various levels of post-acute care while they are working to regain independence and function. As Figure 46–1 illustrates, the "Journey" involves associate interventions across a number of patient touchpoints throughout their stay. Each of these steps is defined in advance so both the patient and their family/caregivers will know what to expect during the course of the stay at Marianjoy.

Key to the entire approach is the management of expectations for the patient's recovery. This is especially highlighted for staff during team meetings and discharge planning discussions with the patient and their family/caregiver. At each step of the "Journey," associate attention is focused on the importance of service excellence in the provision of care. Patient satisfaction outcomes are consistently discussed and disseminated across leadership teams and at department staff meetings. Patients also receive a postdischarge follow-up call process to ensure adherence to discharge plans and to address any concerns related to the various level of care transitions. This proactive service recovery and repair strategy has identified a number of areas for ongoing process improvement at Marianjoy.

Results

To date this service excellence strategy has exceeded expectations. Overall patient satisfaction rose to the 81st percentile of the all-hospital Press Ganey Database in fiscal year (FY) 2010 and the 86th percentile in FY 2011. When compared to other free-standing rehabilitation facilities in the same database, patient satisfaction reached the 90th percentile in FY 2010 and the 95th in FY 2011. Overall discharge specific scores increased to the 75th and 84th percentiles, respectively, during those same time periods. These achievements were recognized locally by the Illinois Hospital Association (IHA) in 2011. Marianjoy was the recipient of the first annual Innovation in Quality Award for Specialty Hospitals from the IHA acknowledging outstanding quality improvement programs that focus on better patient care and outcomes.

Next Steps

This organizationwide initiative demonstrated to leaders and associates alike the depth of the team's capacity and power to innovate and change practices to affect patient satisfaction and improve patient transitions across the continuum of post-acute care. In spite of the success achieved to date, members of the organization have not rested on the initial improvement achieved through the implementation of the "Journey." In early FY 2012, the Service Excellence team actively sought feedback from current and past patients to enhance and revise the "Journey" so that it can continue to evolve and meet the ever-changing needs of the post-acute care environment. The flexible nature of the process will ensure that patients will continue to understand how they will be navigating the complex transitions of care that occur in the post-acute care setting, as well as be satisfied with the excellent service provided by the clinical, therapy, and ancillary support services associates of Marianjoy.

Discussion Questions

1. Why was this initiative so important to the leadership of Marianjoy?

2. What organizational factors contributed to the organization's success?

3. What features of the "Journey" do you consider to be most beneficial?

4. How might the "Journey" be adapted to better meet the needs of patients and family/caregivers at Marianjoy?

5. What characteristics made the Service Excellence team successful?

Group Exercise

What would a similar "Journey" look like in an:

- Acute inpatient setting
- Outpatient clinic
- Ambulatory surgery setting

Case 47

Team Collaboration in Delivering Integrated Systems of Care

CASE CONTRIBUTOR Ben Spedding

Situation

As vice president of Business Development for a regional nonprofit behavioral health services provider (BHS) in Central New Jersey, Stewart was often in the position to talk to clients (including health insurance plans and large employer groups) about what types of clinical programs they wanted. For instance, health insurance plans were looking for clinical programs that focused on stabilization and referral to qualified outpatient programs instead of extended stays in a hospital inpatient unit. Stewart would then meet with his clinical and financial directors at BHS to determine whether or not they could accommodate the requests, and if so, they would work out the details (such as write job descriptions, determine costs and charges, access points, and clinical processes).

BHS had a long-standing reputation in the market for prudent and meaningful collection of utilization and outcomes data on services provided to their clients. Given this reputation, BHS's clinical programs were highly regarded and the agency held many current state and national certifications, including from the Joint Commission and the National Committee for Quality Assurance (NCQA). As a result, they had the opportunity to venture into new markets as they were well positioned with their current treatment programs. Their intensive outpatient treatment program (IOP), for example, was offered to clients in lieu of hospitalization and they were able to negotiate reimbursement payment on a case rate basis versus fee-for-service charges. This reimbursement method provided BHS with more money and freedom up front to determine treatment options, but it required a different level of utilization management (UM) from their standard retroactive UM, such as quality measures including patient satisfaction assessed at discharge. It also required a team approach to an outpatient clinical focus, which meant that once consumers of the IOP were stabilized and returned to a supportive living environment, the outpatient clinician assigned to the treatment needed to work directly with BHS's UM department to determine a treatment plan. This plan would be patient centered while at the same time maximize the case rate payment. In other words, high-quality, cost-effective services needed to be delivered adequately and efficiently, but no more and no less.

Stewart's job responsibilities transitioned from building the network, which involved recruiting, interviewing, and contracting requirements, to leading contracted clinicians through the administrative and clinical management issues required on each new contract. More than once he found himself backed up against the wall by a hostile group of newly minted network providers. Stewart found that only through numerous training meetings and one-on-one sessions on the phone or in person did he begin to get a better sense of where they stood regarding managed care, team collaboration on treatment planning, and receptivity to intrusions into the "art" of their practice. Most were not at all prepared to follow collaborative treatment planning process recommendations based on proactive UM and clinical best practices. Instead, as private practitioners they expected to negotiate a certain number of approved treatment sessions with the payor, regardless of the patient's progress throughout the treatment process. It took well over a year's worth of training and network meetings in order to develop the relationships required to create the level of collaboration necessary for clinical success and prepare BHS to move forward into the next level of contracting relationships. These new contracts included broader case rate and subcapitated types of payment arrangements.

Background

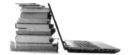

BHS is a large well-respected behavioral health services provider that wanted to develop and extend a more diversified continuum of services to their current clients (the State of New Jersey) as well as to new markets (commercial insurance, Medicare, and private pay). The CEO of BHS understood the company's long-standing commitment to serving the chronically ill population and supporting the idea that their core clinical competencies could be bundled in a way that would be attractive to higher functioning clients, such as the commercially insured. This market expansion opportunity would generate more revenue for BHS, which could then be redirected to enhance infrastructure support systems and clinical programs across the agency. Market changes in behavioral health delivery and payment systems required independent practitioners to develop new skills and knowledge in order to keep their practices viable. As a consequence, they were open to creating new ventures that would allow them to continue in their clinical practices while accessing new market opportunities.

To supplement their continuum of care, BHS expanded its clinician network in part by contracting with private practitioners. These clinicians were selected based upon their location (for ease of consumer access), their various certifications and areas of expertise (along with minimum state and contract licensing standards), and the idea that they were "managed care friendly." As a non-hospital based, private nonprofit organization, BHS found itself attracting and winning more and more contracts for structured and traditional outpatient type programs, which drove a need for increased capacity. BHS saw this network expansion as a win-win for both the agency and for private practice clinicians. It was a success for the agency because it resulted in seasoned, professional counselors with geographical and clinical diversity. It was also a success for the clinicians as they would gain access to new clients through better system support such as central access, on-call emergency access to a psychiatrist 24/7, and various accreditations/quality processes. The idea of looking for clinicians who were "managed care friendly" simply reflected the reality that some clinicians were in open opposition to the whole notion of participating in a collaborative process with providers, such as BHS, in deciding the "who," "what," "when," and "how long" of a therapeutic process. Adding clinicians to the network who were unfavorable to managed care could cause training and administrative obstacles. Therefore, Stewart had to establish rigorous guidelines for an internal selection and certification process for potential new clinicians.

Next Steps

Given these challenges, executive management asked Stewart to determine the best way in which to formalize the selection, training, and certification process for newly contracted clinicians with BHS.

Discussion Questions

1. What leadership issues will Stewart face in organizing the private practice clinicians into a collaborative team?

2. How will the clinicians' values and/or opinions factor into their acceptance of the clinical management process followed by BHS?

3. Discuss the importance of communication and training in the process of building the acceptance and collaboration of new network providers.

4. Identify what you believe to be representative traits for team collaboration. How would you prioritize and incorporate them into guidelines to use for building a collaborative clinical team?

5. Discuss the important issues around reimbursement, referral, and practice patterns that providers and health insurance plans must consider when negotiating a network agreement.

Case 48

CASE CONTRIBUTOR Deymon X. Fleming

Situation

Jorge, the Syphilis Elimination Coordinator for the Puerto Rico Department of Health (PRDOH), reviewed his local response plan developed by the PRDOH to respond to a recent syphilis outbreak in Puerto Rico. Reports from the surveillance unit indicated that there was an increase of 33.0% of primary and secondary syphilis in the recent year over the prior year. Fifty-four percent of the cases were males and 46% were females. The 30–39 age demographic accounted for the highest percentage of all cases, 34.2%.

In developing the local response plan, Jorge drew on his experiences from the outbreak in 2001 in Mayaguez, Puerto Rico. This outbreak occurred during January through March 2001. A total of 16 early syphilis cases (six primary, five secondary, five early latent) were reported, representing a 78% increase over the same time period in 2000. An outbreak response team consisting of 21 people was deployed to the area for two weeks in March. Screenings were done in the area, resulting in 123 tests performed. Ten cases of infectious syphilis were detected and treated. An analysis of the outbreak revealed risk factors of sex workers and drug use. The supervisor submitted a report of the outbreak and performed an evaluation of what resources would be needed in a future outbreak. Additional resources recommended were more nurses and doctors on the outbreak response team and more government vehicles.

Jorge's job is to streamline departmental activities to address the most urgent situations, such as congenital syphilis and outbreaks. The PRDOH has developed and implemented detailed collaborative and contractual agreements that outline the expectations for service provision. In order to be successful, Jorge recognizes that collaborations with current community-based organizations must be well planned and benefit diverse populations including youth, sex workers, substance abusers, and other high-risk populations. In responding to this latest outbreak, Jorge will need to enlist members of the community to assist in the planning and coordinating of syphilis elimination activities. Moreover, he will need to obtain technical assistance in planning and developing strategies to engage members of civic organizations and policy makers. Jorge also understands the importance of bridging the gap between contracted service providers and the PRDOH. He will need to consider methods to provide Disease Intervention Specialist (DIS) training to appropriate healthcare agencies, and allow the contracted service providers to test and follow up positive syphilis cases and patient sex partners in accordance with Sexually Transmitted Disease (STD) Program standards and supervision. Jorge has determined that it is absolutely critical that he dedicate and maintain a mobile van for the exclusive use of community-based syphilis elimination activities.

Background

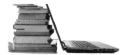

In 1994, health care for Puerto Rico's medically indigent population, defined as <200% of the Commonwealth poverty level ($8,200 for a family of four), shifted from a public healthcare system to a Medicaid managed care system, known as Reforma. Under the public healthcare system, the PRDOH provided medical care through a system of public hospitals and clinics. Legislation created the Puerto Rico Health Insurance Administration (ASES) to contract with managed care organizations (MCOs) to provide quality medical and hospital care to the residents of Puerto Rico regardless of ability to pay. It is unclear if this change to a Medicaid managed care system contributed to the outbreak; however, anecdotally one could deduce that having more access to medical services would provide better opportunity to detect disease.

The PRDOH along with recommendations from the U.S. Centers for Disease Control and Prevention determine when a disease is an outbreak and when there is a need for a response. The threshold for declaring an outbreak is a 10% increase in cases as compared to the same time period over the previous year. However, surveillance does not routinely analyze data to determine if an increase is occurring. Instead, a DIS in an area may notice that he or she is seeing more cases of a particular disease than usual. The DIS will notify his or her supervisor, who will then notify the Syphilis Elimination Coordinator. The coordinator will request that surveillance analyze the data for the time period and compare it to the previous year. The STD program will look at the criteria used to define the threshold for declaring an outbreak and revise the criteria. For example, by using a 10% increase in cases as the threshold, a rise in cases from one to three, or even one to two, would trigger a response when in fact there may be no outbreak at all. Moreover, if social and behavioral factors are not considered, an outbreak may be missed. For example, there could be a significant rise in cases among groups such as men having sex with men, which would not total a 10% increase in total cases.

An outbreak response team consists of the Syphilis Elimination Coordinator, Syphilis Elimination Team DIS, local area DIS, medical services person, and local area nurses. All supplies are sent to the area from San Juan. Local participation in the outbreak response is coordinated by the Syphilis Elimination Coordinator. However, this is done as the outbreak is happening, as it is not previously arranged. The STD program should involve the local community in the planning of an outbreak response before the outbreak occurs. Agreements are made with local community-based organizations (CBOs) and medical facilities to provide personnel and supplies if needed.

Next Steps

As Jorge considers what steps to take to implement the outbreak response, he needs to be mindful of important considerations. First, there is limited dissemination of information to local partners and no media involvement. The program coordinators feel that if the media is informed of an outbreak, they will send reporters, and sensationalize the facts. Instead, information is given to the local area DIS and director, and is presented at conferences.

Second, Jorge, in his supervisory role, needs to recommend resources that might be required in the future. Third, the response plan is reactive instead of proactive, and as such does not implement efforts to evaluate how the response affects the disease in the community. Fourth, the written outbreak response plan is known to employees in the San Juan area, but is not shared with other regions. The outbreak response is handled by San Juan with input from the local area. Considering these factors, Jorge wonders if the program that attempts to prevent future outbreaks by performing screenings in local areas and providing STD education covers all bases effectively.

Discussion Questions

1. Who are the appropriate partners Jorge should involve in an outbreak response plan?

2. Are the assessment methods for declaring an outbreak adequate?

3. How should the plan be disseminated and communicated to partners?

4. Are the plans for outbreak prevention too reactive? What proactive measures would you recommend?

Case 49

Pacific Needle Exchange Program

CASE CONTRIBUTOR **James Allen Johnson, III**

Situation

Pacific Needle Exchange (PNEX), a one-for-one syringe exchange program funded by the Hawaii Department of Health, is a nonprofit organization dedicated to the reduction of HIV prevalence amongst injection drug users (IDU) in the state of Hawaii. PNEX provides hypodermic syringes to IDUs through a one-for-one exchange (one new syringe is provided for every used syringe discarded at a designated PNEX exchange location) along with condoms and health education materials relevant to that particular population. PNEX was established in 1989 and has been successful in reducing the prevalence of HIV within Hawaii's IDU population from around 50% in 1989 to around 1.5% where it has persisted since 2001. PNEX is regarded nationally as a success and has served as a model for emerging syringe exchange programs in other states.

Stephen Maturin, MPH, the executive director of PNEX, received the annual report on the status of the IDU population it serves. Because of the program's success in reducing the spread of HIV, Mr. Maturin decided to include a study on the prevalence of hepatitis C virus (HCV), a virus that commonly affects IDUs, in this year's annual report. He was particularly concerned by the results of the HCV study, which indicated that 87% of the IDU population PNEX serves tested positive for HCV antigens.

Background

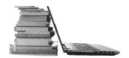

HCV typically has a higher prevalence in IDU populations than does HIV. One explanation for this may be that HCV has the ability to survive outside of the body while HIV typically cannot. Because hypodermic syringes form a semi-vacuum environment, HIV can survive in a syringe long enough to potentially infect another person if the syringe is reused and not properly sterilized. Outside of syringes or the human body, there are few known places HIV can survive, limiting its spread to the exchange of fluids through sexual intercourse and blood-to-blood contact (which occurs with the reuse of infected syringes). Like HIV, HCV is a blood-borne pathogen but, unlike HIV, it can survive outside the body. Because of this, unlike HIV, HCV can be transmitted via a material medium. In the case of IDUs, this medium is often "cookers" (tools such as spoons, miniature medal cups, etc. used to prepare drugs through the process of heating), tourniquets, and pieces of cotton used in the injection process. Because HCV can survive outside of the body on inanimate objects, it can spread when these objects are shared. Such is the case when two or more people reusing their own syringes (not directly sharing) draw from the same "cooker." If one person in the group sharing the "cooker" has HCV, everyone has been exposed to the virus, potentially becoming infected. This exposure happened despite taking some of the necessary precautions to avoid HIV exposure (not sharing used syringes).

Next Steps

The following week Stephen called a meeting with the outreach workers to discuss the findings of the study and their possible implications. During the meeting, he will discuss his goal to reduce the prevalence of HCV by half over the next 10 years. Stephen plans to ask his team to suggest changes to the needle exchange program necessary to achieve this goal while maintaining the successful campaign against the spread of HIV.

Discussion Questions

1. With a grant from the Department of Health to address HCV, what strategies should the outreach workers recommend?

2. What are some of the possible challenges of addressing the HCV epidemic in an IDU population?

3. One can be infected with HCV for 20 or more years before symptoms begin to appear. What unique challenges may this present and how could they be overcome?

Case 50

Post-EHR Implementation—The Recovery Room Slowdown

CASE CONTRIBUTOR Genesa L. Mays

Situation

At Winston Bay Medical Center ("Winston Bay"), Christina Dash is the director of the postanesthesia recovery room ("recovery room"). She is known for her satisfactory completion of initiatives and directives. Her clinical outcomes, partnership with surgeons, and satisfaction scores have increased in the last two years. Her clinical staff is culturally diverse and the average turnover rate is less than 5%. Clinical supervisors are staffed one per shift and the patient to staff ratio is 2:1. This ratio changes to 1:1 when the unit receives a trauma, transplant, or medically unstable patient.

An electronic health record (EHR) has been implemented in the recovery room. One of the objectives of the implementation will be to capture clinical data that are necessary for quality improvement. Financial data will not be captured in the EHR and are being manually entered on logs that are stored for about eight years. This storage requirement is for regulatory purposes. The nurses are working hard to input clinical data into the new EHR. However, the average patient recovery time has increased by more than 30% due to the nurses having difficulty in entering data into the EHR. Management predicted an increase in recovery service time during the EHR implementation, but was optimistic that the trend would decrease in a few weeks. After two months, however, the learning curve continued and the recovery nurses were still having difficulty.

As a result of the EHR input difficulty, delays in transporting patients from the surgical suite to the recovery room have been reported. Surgeons are extremely upset about the delay and maintain cautious concern over patient safety. The average delay time is 30 to 95 minutes. Surgical nurses document the delays in a multifunctional software system that captures data for both clinical and financial purposes. (This system is separate from the newly implemented EHR.) First cases are starting on time and entering the recovery room within timely parameters. About 40% of the cases following the first cases, however, are delayed entry into the recovery room. Performance indicators have been showing unfavorable results. Declining staff productivity for both the recovery room and the surgical area is one of the unfavorable performance outcomes. Current staff productivity rate is 75% compared to the target percentage of 95%. Productivity is measured by patient volume and the number of staff-worked hours. Despite the declining volume, staffing patterns for both units have remained unchanged.

The Surgical Services Department is managed by Steven Carter. Over the past two years, the patient volume within the Surgical Services Department has declined by more than 22%. All surgical specialties have declined. Orthopedic and spine surgeries have declined by more than 25% and these service lines are responsible for generating more than 40% of the gross revenue for the perioperative service line. If the current trends of patient volume continue, profit margins will decline rapidly.

With declining profits, volume, surgeon satisfaction rates, productivity targets, and increasing payroll spending, executive leadership is demanding an immediate resolution. An impromptu meeting has been called with departmental leadership. All management staff, including Christina, enters the conference room for a scheduled two-hour meeting. In the conference room at Winston Bay, the facility's president, chief financial officer, and vice presidents are in attendance. Direct leadership has been given one month to change the present trends and outcomes.

Background

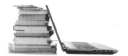

Winston Bay is located in the center of a major metropolitan city that has a population of 6.5 million. The flagship site has over 700 beds with an average occupancy rate of 71% and is a Level I trauma system. The system has been recognized for numerous achievements in service and quality outcomes. More than 15 affiliates within the system are strategic, situated across the urban and rural areas of the county. The healthcare system resides in a non-certificate of need (CON) state. Within the last eight months, more than four competing entities have been constructed. One of the competing entities is a physician partnership site for orthopedic and spine surgery.

Christina and the Surgical Services directors have access to a Business Intelligence (BI) team of skilled workers. The BI department is uniquely staffed with technical report writers and other technical disciplines. The primary duty of the team is to provide statistical reporting for departmental management. The BI team is supervised by a financial director who has more than 20 years of experience. The BI team is tasked with producing reports and other analytic information for the leadership team. Information is easily retrieved from the Surgical Services' software systems. Financial information for the recovery room exists on paper logs and is not easily retrievable. The BI staff must enter financial data from the log into an electronic format for data disclosure. Additionally, historical clinical data for the recovery room cannot be retrieved from the newly implemented EHR system. Winston Bay's information systems department is addressing the clinical issue. However, the problem in gathering clinical data from the EHR will not be resolved for another three months.

Next Steps

The vice president of Clinical Operations of Winston Bay schedules a meeting with Christina and Steven to discuss concerns with the recent surgical and recovery activities. Leadership must disclose a plan of action within two weeks.

Discussion Questions

1. How should the leadership team develop a plan to address the declining performance measures?

2. What data requirements will be needed to make informed decisions?

3. Identify the clinical and financial data requirements for the recovery room. How will the data be extracted and used to improve outcomes for the recovery room? Should there be any data requirements for the Surgical Services Department? Explain.

4. What data requirements are needed to improve the staff productivity of the surgical services and the recovery room?

5. Why are performance indicators important and how should they be used to support decision making?

6. How often should performance indicator data be reported and used for management purposes?

Case 51

Go or No Go—An Executive's Information System Dilemma

CASE CONTRIBUTOR Margaret Ozan Rafferty

Situation

Walking up the stairs to the executive meeting rooms, Senior Vice President Susan Boscarino felt a chill in the fall air and a familiar twinge in her stomach. She was heading to the weekly Great Lakes Health senior team meeting where she anticipated another round of heated discussions with her peers about the installation of the new information system platform. Susan knew this would be a tough meeting as they would vote on whether or not to continue with the installation.

Background

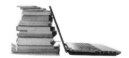

Susan was the newest member of the executive team at Great Lakes Health, a unionized two-hospital system with revenues of $550 million located in the Midwest. The rest of the group had been at the organization for over two years. Four members of the team had worked together in a previous organization where their four-hospital system became the market leader. Believing they could duplicate their success by "turning Great Lakes Health around," the team had realigned the organization's finances by reducing expenses, proposing several service line consolidations, and addressing many quality improvement issues. The CEO's vision was to position Great Lakes Health as the premier provider of health care for the southeast corner of the state. The team knew this was going to be a huge challenge as the local population was declining, and more and more people in the service area were traveling 30 miles to the east to the university hospitals in the major metropolitan area for their health care. A strategic plan with financial projections was developed that outlined aggressive goals for the next four years.

Susan joined the organization two months ago bringing a strong background in clinical and operations performance as well as a passion for employee and patient engagement. During the hiring process, she was wooed by the executive search firm and the Great Lakes Health executive team, which presented a sound financial plan and a sense of camaraderie that appealed to her. She was also impressed that so many members of the Great Lakes Health team had followed the CEO, Thomas Hurd, from their previous organization.

Late last year, with the feeling that most of the financial losses were averted, the organization embarked on the quest to update its antiquated information system. The existing information system was installed in the early 1980s and although Great Lakes Health received regular software updates from its long-term vendor, the information technology (IT) system had become obsolete. The old system lacked the ability to fully integrate with the hospital's financial platform and was unable to handle diagnostic code integration or meet the documentation needs of the hospitals. The leadership knew it needed to continue to reduce costs and improve care, and after some analysis decided to move forward with an investment in a new information system.

Susan knew this project's effect on the budget was significant and that the organization needed to align the interests of its administrators, clinicians, and IT experts. From her previous IT project experience, she knew the importance of a clearly communicated budget with key milestones and strong project leadership. She also recognized the importance of employee participation in creating buy-in, commitment, and a sense of ownership. Susan knew that staff and users with interest and expertise in information systems should be assigned to the implementation teams. Their input would be needed to resolve implementation-related conflicts. In addition, Susan understood that organizations needed to analyze the trade-offs between purchasing the best-of-the-best system and the appropriate choice for the organization based on the hospital's overall objectives, time frames, and funds. Being a systems thinker, Susan knew it was important to consider the interconnectivity and complexity of the organization.

As Great Lakes Health lacked a chief information officer (CIO), Peter Clarke, vice president of Marketing, was named to lead the initiative. What Peter lacked in IT experience, he made up for in enthusiasm. Once the decision was made to explore options for a new system, Peter and the IT team promptly sent out a request for proposal (RFP) to leading vendors. Under Peter's leadership, there were discussions with the medical staff leadership during the vendor selection process. Many vendors came to Great Lakes Health and gave lengthy presentations to the executive team and medical staff. Frontline staff and managers from across the hospital system were involved in the vendor selection process. The vendor Venus Systems was eventually selected by the senior team, with a very strong recommendation from the medical executive staff.

Venus was known as the "gold standard" of IT in the healthcare industry. Its clients consisted of over 100 large hospitals and academic medical centers, and the company had over $1 billion in revenues the previous year. The total cost of the system installation was projected at $85 million, with ongoing maintenance fees of approximately 26% of the license fee. Great Lakes Health's leadership team decided to make the additional investment needed to go with this high-priced vendor. According to the CEO, "We need a world-class system to help make us a world-class organization." They based their decision primarily on projected savings from reductions in medical errors and anticipated improvements in financial metrics including bill collections. Based on these forecasts, the system was projected to break even at the end of year four.

After the nonrefundable down payment of $26 million was made, installation of the system began. Peter began recruiting additional IT experts necessary to start up the project. He quickly found that IT professionals were not that eager to move to the Midwest. Peter also realized that the salaries he had budgeted for these new positions were too low and did not match the compensation packages offered by organizations in the metro area just

35 miles away. As a result, Peter had to offer his candidates higher salaries, which made a significant dent in his expense forecast and upset many existing employees who also demanded the same level of compensation. The delay in finding qualified staff hampered the implementation timeline, resulting in additional costs.

Employees enjoyed some of the early modules of the Venus system rollout, including the order entry platform, staff email capabilities, and new terminals. Case management implemented several new tracks focused on high-volume DRGs, and soon lengths of stay started to reduce. Three new physician groups joined the organization. Most members of these groups cited the physician-friendly Venus system as a key recruitment factor.

By the end of the summer, an additional $9 million was invested in the Venus installation. However, during that time Great Lakes Health's financial situation began to deteriorate. Previous savings gained through restructuring were not sustainable as many departing core staff were replaced with overtime and high-priced agency hires. Accounts receivable days inched back up from a low of 52 to over 100 days. An anticipated $5 million payment by the government to Great Lakes Health as a disproportionate share hospital (DSH) was postponed for another 15 months, sending the fiscal year's budget into a tailspin. The planned closing of services at one of the hospital's campuses was met with fierce resistance from community leaders forcing the hospital to continue to provide these services at a significant loss for the organization. A large physician group decided at the last minute that they were not going to relocate to the Great Lakes Health's newly built medical office building, leaving over two floors of office space without tenants and lease income. Day's cash on hand became so critical that the CFO's team privately joked it was often "hour's cash on hand." In addition, a patient occurrence at one of the hospital's emergency rooms raised a red flag with the Joint Commission and the local public health authorities. As a result, these organizations now made frequent unannounced visits to the campuses, resulting in multiple warnings and concerns of a loss of accreditation.

Next Steps

Susan pondered all these issues as she entered the meeting room. The team was going to vote today on whether to move forward with the rest of the Venus installation or to absorb the sunk costs to date and table implementation of the project. The physicians had lobbied the team not to stop the installation. Catching wind of the discussion, some employees threatened to strike if the organization returned to the old system. The executive team had to make a decision on the Venus system. Moving forward to continue funding the project meant taking resources from Great Lakes Health's reserves. Stopping meant no additional payments to Venus, helping the bottom line but losing the investment made to date as well as the order entry platform and returning to the old system. Based on last week's conversations, Susan knew the vote was split among her peers on the seven-member team. She would cast the deciding vote—move forward or stop the install.

Discussion Questions

1. What did the executive team do successfully and not so successfully in the initial stages of the information system evaluation and installation project?

2. What are the primary factors that led to this decision point for Great Lakes Health? Was it the result of poor planning?

3. Should Great Lakes Health have initiated a major IT project without an experienced CIO? Why or why not?

4. Discuss the likely reactions of stakeholders to a vote to move forward and a vote to stop the install. How should the executive team consider these reactions in deciding their votes?

5. What are the implications for Great Lakes Health if it decides not to proceed with the install?

6. What should Susan do?

Case 52

CASE CONTRIBUTOR Anthony Drautz

Situation

To address the issue of ever-increasing demands on minimum program requirements, contractual obligations, and heightened public expectation, a large local health department's (LHD) Environmental Health Services (EHS) unit needed to implement an electronic permitting, inspection, document generation, storage, reporting, and management tool. The LHD has had to do "more with less" in recent years. After review of multiple electronic environmental health management software packages, Luke, the EHS administrator, was determined that the internal creation of this type of system would be best suited to meet the minimum program requirements and goals of the department. Luke and his staff partnered with the county's Department of Information Technology, creating a team that developed an integrated, web-based, electronic inspection and permitting system. The system has modules that allow for the administration and management of multiple environmental health programs, including food safety, food service management certification, water well permitting and inspection, onsite sewage disposal system permitting and inspection, nuisance complaint investigations, and the public health water testing laboratory.

The overall goal of the team was to provide an easy-to-use, flexible tool that allows for the permitting, inspection, and investigation of multiple environmental health programs. Enhanced access to records, the ability to schedule daily activities and generate a workload management report to improve the flow of work through OCHD were also critical components that were recognized by Luke as necessary for the success of the electronic system. The scheduling and workload management system tool modules could be used by every role within EHS that contributes to the flow of work through the department. The team's solution had to promote teamwork through enhanced access to records within and across roles, as well as provide administration with the necessary information to make informed decisions regarding program and resource management, workload assignments, geographic designations, and investigation resolution. Accountability and efficiency of Luke's staff and quality of service and records generated from the electronic system would also be enhanced and improved. The projected return on investment was also critical in securing funding and support from elected officials and county administration.

Background

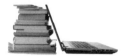

The LHD is located in the Midwest and serves one of largest populations in the state. The county comprises numerous independent cities, villages, and townships. With a mix of urban and rural communities, the county offers a variety of residential and business settings to a diverse, affluent, and educated population demographic. The county ranks as one of the wealthiest in the nation among counties with populations of more than one million people. A high tech corridor is headquartered in the county, which greatly impacts the promotion and development of advanced technology in the region. The county is home to approximately 42,000 businesses, including many foreign-owned companies. There are over 30 universities, colleges, and technical schools. The population has grown consistently every year since 2000. The median household income far exceeds the national average. The county's strong economic base and progressive infrastructure continues to offer its citizens the opportunity to prosper. The county has a largely affluent, educated population demographic that embraces and supports the use of technology such as an electronic management tool.

The LHD is the largest local health department in the state. Within the LHD, the EHS unit is administered out of three regional offices led by an administrator, two program chiefs, seven field supervisors, and 58 public health sanitarians. The administrator, chiefs, and supervisors all have master's level degrees and are registered sanitarians (RSs) in the state or registered environmental health specialists (REHSs) with the National Environmental Health Association (NEHA). Included in the group of 58 sanitarians are 24 senior sanitarians, who are registered sanitarians that may assist and mentor less experienced or credentialed staff. Their expertise and leadership has been invaluable in the implementation of the electronic system.

Each office is responsible for all environmental health programs in their respective geographic areas. Luke's staff has been assigned tablet computers, mobile printers, global positioning system (GPS) units, and wireless Internet capabilities in order to complete program assignments through the electronic system. The change to a paperless work environment proved to be a particular challenge for many of Luke's field staff and supervisors. Orientation to the use of advanced technology was met with resistance by some that feared the change and were not technologically savvy. Luke ensured that his staff was continuously trained as the phased implementation of the electronic system progressed over a three-year period. System module pilot groups and focus group environments were created to discuss system "bugs" and to make recommendations for enhancements to the system to improve functionality and the end product. These opportunities have softened the shock of the change in business practices and reorganization of the unit.

Next Steps

The State Department of Agriculture (SDA) recently decided to proceed with an electronic licensing and permitting system for their retail food service program. Their review of the multiple available products on the market resulted in the SDA selection of the county's electronic system to be used statewide by SDA food safety inspectors. The county provided the program to SDA at no cost. In turn, the SDA and State Department of Information Technology are in the process of modifying the system to release and support the electronic system for other local health departments in the state. This will improve the food safety program and consistency in the administration of the program statewide.

The LHD continues to make enhancements to the electronic system and expand the capabilities of its use. Water well and onsite sewage disposal system locations are captured using GPS. Drinking water test results are also entered into the system. This data can be reported, tracked, and mapped through geographic information system (GIS) software for spatial analysis of emerging issues, epidemiological investigations, and program management by Luke and other unit administrators in the LHD. The comprehensive use of GIS technology is an integral component of the electronic system.

The focus groups and training opportunities have continued to relax the apprehension of staff that found the change to the electronic environment a challenge. Luke and his staff have realized numerous benefits from this initiative. Staff productivity and quality of work are measurable outcomes that have proven the success of the implementation of an electronic management system. Compliance with state-mandated minimum program requirements, periodic reporting requirements, and contractual obligations of all environmental health programs have improved. The LHD has been recognized by state agencies and national organizations for the development and implementation of this cutting edge technology, including the accreditation with commendation by the SDA, Department of Community Health, and the Department of Environmental Quality.

Discussion Questions

1. How can the use of electronic management tools improve the quality of records and services, efficiency, and accountability for a regulatory agency such as an environmental health unit in a local health department?

2. Describe a scenario(s) in which the data captured and retrieved from an electronic program management system can be used to recognize emerging issues in environmental health and to assist in epidemiological investigations such as foodborne or waterborne disease outbreaks.

3. Luke experienced some reluctance on the part of staff to accept new technology. What are the challenges of the implementation of advanced technology on program staff?

4. How can an administration effectively manage a smooth transition in business practices to gain staff "buy-in" and acceptance of the change?

Case 53

CASE CONTRIBUTOR **James E. Selby, Jr.**

Situation

The office of pharmaceuticals and biotechnology sciences (OPBS) of the Food and Drug Administration (FDA) is the largest laboratory-based operating office within the FDA. With a combined budget of almost $100 million shared between five operating offices of OPBS, a significant portion of the center for drugs and regulatory evidence (CDRE) budget, it is essential that OPBS has a budget tracking system in place so that they can accurately account for their expenditures. One of the challenges among the five offices of OPBS is that they all have their own method of tracking their budgets. Some of these offices use Excel spreadsheets to track their budgets while others use simple budget databases. Because of this, OPBS as a whole has always either underspent or overspent in previous fiscal years and has never been able to accurately track their budgets.

Every fiscal year, OPBS has many problems in trying to track their expenditures. Complaints on the amount of errors in their expenditure reporting, duplication of efforts in trying to reconcile purchases and expenses as well as even the loss of financial transactions all occur because of a lack of a centralized budget tracking system. Since every office in OPBS tracks their expenditures differently, OPBS is having extreme difficulty in reporting their overall financial status to their center and to the FDA. Pressure is now being put on CDRE from the FDA to better account for their expenditures. Since OPBS has the largest portion of CDRE's budget, OPBS is now being pressured to more accurately account for their expenditures in the new fiscal year. OPBS believes that with a more centralized budget tracking system it will be able to accurately account for the budget in each office as well as track the budget for OPBS as a whole.

After meeting about the need for a more accurate budget tracking system, the senior administrators for each of the offices of OPBS formed a budget system development team in order to develop a system that can accurately track the budget for each office and be able to produce reports on the budget for OPBS. Some of the main issues that the budget system development team feels the new budget tracking system should possess include an ability to produce reports that can account for every line item of OPBS' budget, an ability to reconcile every type of expenditure to include credit card purchases, grants, procurement charges, contracts expenses, and future expenditures that may need to be monitored.

Background

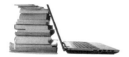

Because of the need to reduce the deficit in the United States, many areas of the government are now being charged with finding ways to reduce their spending. Concerns for the overall fiscal health of the U.S. economy from organizations like the Committee for a Responsible Federal Budget (CRFB) also are voicing their views about the need for a reduction in federal spending. "The country is running out of time to begin addressing its unsustainable fiscal path on its own terms."[1] According to the CRFB, "what the country needs is not deficit reduction just for the sake of deficit reduction. Restructuring our tax and entitlement systems and our discretionary spending programs offers us the chance to make them more efficient at promoting economic growth and saving money."[1] In finalizing the federal budget for the present year, the budget will incorporate a three-year nonsecurity discretionary freeze that will save $250 billion over the next decade. An overall cap on nonsecurity discretionary funding in which key investments are expanded but cutbacks on programs that are ineffective, duplicative, or just wasteful will occur.[2]

Among many government programs that are being asked to review their programs and identify areas that they could reduce their budget, the FDA has been asked to reduce their budget by $77 million. Overall, the budget of the FDA is $8.2 billion so a reduction of $77 million is significant. FDA officials reviewed their financial reports and determined the first way to go about looking for areas that can be financially reduced is to ask each of their centers to do a six-month review on their expenditures starting at the beginning of the calendar year. CDRE asked OPBS to account for their expenditures and provide a six-month report on its financial status. As the largest office with the biggest portion of CDRE's budget, it is critically important that OPBS accurately accounts for their expenditures; thus, the need for a system that can track and report their expenditures is critical.

Next Steps

The budget system development team needs to create a budget tracking system that will accurately track the expenditures of each office of OPBS and OPBS as a whole. The team needs to decide what functions are important for the budget tracking system and also what type of program should be used to develop the system. Since the senior administrators need to begin tracking their budgets and produce an accurate account for CDRE by the end of the six-month review period, the budget development tracking system needs to be created expeditiously. The team has also been asked to present the financial status of OPBS using the new budget tracking system that they develop.

Note: OPBS and CDRE are fictional divisions within the FDA created for illustrative purposes.

Discussion Questions

1. What issues do you think the team of senior administrators will face when trying to develop a unified budget tracking system since they have used different methods in the past to track the budgets within their respective offices?

2. Please discuss the pros and cons of working as a team in developing this unified budget tracking system.

3. If you were a senior administrator on this team, how would you be able to convince the other senior administrators that the budget tracking system should consist of the budget functions that you believe are important?

4. Please explain how the development of a unified budget tracking system improves public health program management.

References

[1] Committee for a Responsible Federal Budget. (2011). *What we'd like to see in the president's FY2012 budget.* Retrieved from http://crfb.org/sites/default/files/What_Wed_Like_to_See_in_the_Presidents_FY2012_Budget.pdf

[2] Orszag, P. (2010). *Introducing the FY2011 budget.* Retrieved from http://www.whitehouse.gov/omb/blog/10/02/01/Introducing-the-2011-Budget/

Case 54

CASE CONTRIBUTOR **Judy S. Cash**

Situation

Monday had been a difficult day. Another respiratory depression incident had occurred on the orthopedic floor, but this time the patient expired. Clare Rodriquez, the manager of the postanesthesia care unit (PACU) at Talbot Medical Center (Talbot), knew she had to take action so this would never happen again. As she pored over the chart, she reviewed the last 14 hours of this man's life. Mr. Hollis Franks was overweight, had a history of hypertension, and was a loud snorer according to his wife. He had a knee replacement at 7:00 a.m. Monday morning and was rolled into the PACU by 8:30 a.m. reporting pain at a 9. This 76-year old man received intravenous (IV) opioids until his reported pain was a 5. At that time, he was sent to the floor on a patient-controlled analgesia (PCA) pump with morphine available every six minutes with no lockout. The orthopedic nurse reported he arrived to his room nauseated and reporting pain at 7 after the elevator ride and the long trip to his room. The nurse checked to see what medications his surgeon had ordered and gave him some Phenergan for nausea and a muscle relaxant pill for his pain since he already had the morphine pump. His wife said he continued to push his pain pump button so he wouldn't hurt, but fell asleep while talking to her. She was concerned about this behavior and asked his nurse if this was normal. The nurse asked if he had slept well the night before and his wife said no. The nurse told the wife he was probably just now getting comfortable and would benefit from the rest. His wife of 54 years sat with him while he slept. She didn't notice his shallow breathing. She didn't want the pain to wake him up, so every time she thought about it, she would push his pain button for him so his pain wouldn't return. His wife decided to go home, feed the dogs, and return in the morning. When she tried to rouse him to say good night, he wouldn't wake up. She called the nurse. The nurse called the code team, but it was too late. Mr. Franks had stopped breathing. The code team could not revive him. This was not the first time a patient at Talbot had suffered from respiratory depression, but this was the first death. This sentinel event would change practice at Talbot.

As the manager of the PACU, Clare had been trending data (i.e., collecting the reported pain level for the first 30 minutes on each patient arriving from the operating room into the PACU) on arrival from the operating room (OR) for three months. Her staff had brought this issue to the chief of anesthesiology in hopes of improving anesthesia's pain management coverage intraoperatively. Patients were arriving from the OR reporting their pain as intolerable. The data was showing 54% of the patients were reporting pain at an 8 or more within the first 30 minutes of arriving in the recovery room. The nurses were administrating more morphine, Dilaudid, and fentanyl than previous years and were concerned about overloading these patients with pain medications, especially to those who were overweight.

Clare knew there would be a root cause analysis on this case. She and the manager from the orthopedic floor had been talking about this for the last two months looking for common themes. The orthopedic manager said every adverse incident had involved Phenergan. One of the orthopedic nurses said it seemed that whenever they gave an oral pain medication along with a muscle relaxant and a sleeping pill, the patients became obtunded. The Rapid Response Team (RRT) told them that 20 calls in three months was a red flag. Narcan and applying a rebreather mask had worked in all the other cases. However, it hadn't worked on this Monday. Mr. Franks was dead.

Background

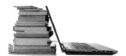

Talbot is a Level 1 trauma center in the heart of a large urban city. Its magnet status and 109-year history as a teaching hospital provides it with much respect and status within the community. Talbot has a strong research practice and is focused on evidence-based patient care. Clare collected the data on pain levels at Talbot to determine if undermedicating by anesthesia providers in the OR was resulting in her nurses overdosing their patients with opioids in the recovery room. She was aware her nurses were using different opioids to treat pain. Her attention, however, was limited to blaming anesthesia for poor pain management. Four months ago, a new contract brought in certified registered nurse anesthetists (CRNAs) to form Anesthesia Care Teams. She immediately noticed a change in pain scores. The CRNAs would use quick-acting, short-life fentanyl rather than longer-acting morphine or Dilaudid. She told the chief of anesthesiology that her nurses had to play "catch up" in treating pain.

Next Steps

After talking to the orthopedic clinical manager, Clare learned that orthopedic nurses also made it a practice to "dabble" in polypharmacy in an effort to ease the pain of surgery. The more they compared notes, the more they saw common themes emerging. The adverse events related to respiratory depression shared these facts: the patients were obese, on PCA pain pumps, all had a history of snoring, and were the recipients of a combination of opioids, muscle relaxants, sedating nausea medicine, and sleeping medications. One of the anesthesia physicians gave them an article on undiagnosed sleep apnea and pulse-ox monitoring devices for surgical patients. The problem was growing more complex the more they researched. The two managers realized this was a much larger problem, and the responsibility was far-reaching. Clare's first priority will be to gather all the facts for the root cause analysis. It will be important to make sure all stakeholders are at the table to address this problem. Clare recognizes that critical to patient safety is developing a plan to protect patients at risk when they come to Talbot for surgery, but how?

Discussion Questions

1. What are the main facts that Clare needs to consider in developing the root cause analysis? What disciplines should be involved?

2. Who is responsible for protecting surgery patients? As an administrator, how do you assess and manage accountability across departments?

3. Identify the larger organizational issues for Talbot to consider in this case.

4. What obligations do hospitals have to screen and protect high-risk patients?

5. When does this protection responsibility begin and when does it end?

Case 55

Unacceptable Backlogs in the Sterile Processing Department

CASE CONTRIBUTOR **Andrea Frederick**

Situation

Carmen Smith, RN, a new supervisor for the Sterile Processing Department (SPD), has just returned to her office after a meeting of the Surgical Services Leadership Team. She is frustrated with the service demands being made of her department from the operating room (OR) staff. There is a high level of dissatisfaction with the SPD's ability to turn around sterile instruments for the OR. Carmen has been working with a process improvement (PI) team to analyze the SPD instrument turnaround problems and the PI team has identified several opportunities to improve turnaround time. Carmen had hoped to find support and constructive suggestions from her colleagues at the leadership meeting, but she received only criticism and disparagement.

Background

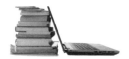

Life in the OR moves at a breakneck pace. Instrument turnaround must be optimized to allow as many procedures as possible each day. SPD efficiency is essential to the success of the OR. The function of the SPD is to create an efficient infrastructure to support the processing of instruments, supplies, and specialty trays for the OR. The SPD must have trained staff, space, processes, and equipment to keep pace with changing instrument types, new guidelines from manufacturers, and infection control guidelines. When the SPD is unable to meet the needs of the OR, the success of the OR is compromised.

The relationship between the SPD and the OR at Central Hospital has been strained for many years. The OR staff has been dissatisfied with the timely availability and quality of surgical instruments from the SPD. This has also been a major source of surgeon dissatisfaction for the organization. The director of surgical services has implemented multiple interventions in the past to try to resolve the long-standing service problem. For instance, the department was recently renovated. Central Hospital administration engaged an outside consultant to develop and implement a redesign of the SPD. The outcome was a much larger cleaning and disinfection area and the implementation of a multiple-cart washer process. When this costly redesign program did not result in improved turnaround, the experienced sterile processing manager was removed and replaced by Carmen. The director of surgical services felt that an RN with direct surgical experience might better understand the service needs of the OR. Carmen has extensive OR experience. She has experience as a circulator, scrub nurse, and first assistant. She felt genuinely respected by the surgeon staff and her OR colleagues until she accepted the SPD supervisory position.

Shortly after taking on the supervisory role, Carmen decided to initiate a PI team to tackle the urgent and increasingly disrespectful service demands from the OR. The team was facilitated by the director of the quality department and included frontline staff from the SPD, OR, and infection control. The team was encouraged to identify everything that they believed contributed to the instrument turnaround problem. No idea was off the table. The team discovered that there were many long-standing, unflattering assumptions held about the SPD. For example, the OR staff felt the SPD staff was lazy and that abuse of the hospital's absenteeism policy contributed to the instrument turnaround problems. The team facilitator insisted that the team objectively and systematically test each theory against available objective data. In their analysis, the team plotted SPD staffing levels against sterile instrument delays in the OR, and no relationship was found. The team then decided to develop a step-by-step process flow for the work performed by the SPD. The drivers and limitations of capacity at each process step were identified. Caseload and instrument demand were detailed out for each day of the week. Patterns emerged. It became clear to the team that Mondays and Wednesdays had the highest case volumes for the OR. These days required the preparation of many complex instrument trays and delivery coordination of loaner trays from multiple outside sources. On Tuesdays and Thursdays, the SPD could not meet the instrument turnaround demand and customer complaints peaked. By overlapping the data, the problem became apparent—steam sterilizer capacity was the bottleneck, not employee work ethic. It was impossible for the steam sterilizer to meet demand during the 16 hours of staffed operation each day.

Next Steps

The team process was helpful in building understanding between the SPD and OR staff. The turnaround pinch point was identified, and now all that was needed was a logical solution. Carmen recognized two viable options. The organization could expand SPD staffing to allow the steam sterilizer to operate 24 hours each day or the organization could purchase a second steam sterilizer and redesign the SPD space once again. When Carmen presented these two options to the Surgical Services Leadership Team, she was reminded that the organization was in the midst of strict cost containment and that no new staff positions could be approved. The team discussion quickly turned back to the old issues of absenteeism and misuse or overuse of short-term disability and Family and Medical Leave Act benefits by the SPD staff.

Despite feeling frustrated and unsupported, Carmen is determined to solve this problem. She has learned exactly how instruments enter the system, are cleaned, packaged, sterilized, and delivered to the OR. She believes the SPD staff is demoralized and that this general perception is contributing to the department's high absenteeism rate. The SPD is critical to the functioning of Central Hospital. Her employees need the respect of their OR colleagues in order for both departments to be effective. Carmen schedules a meeting with the director of quality to discuss next steps.

Discussion Questions

1. How should Carmen move forward to resolve this persistent problem?

2. Did the initial team include all of the necessary stakeholders? What additional team members might you have involved?

3. If you were the director of surgical services, how would you respond to the data analysis developed by the PI team?

4. What other solutions might be available to improve the SPD instrument turnaround time?

5. Describe the challenges of motivating the SPD workforce. What approach would you use to demonstrate the significance of the SPD to the success of every surgical intervention?

Case 56

Responsibility in the Development of a Pressure Ulcer

CASE CONTRIBUTOR Cheryl Daniels

Situation

Stanley George is an 84-year-old male who was admitted to the Dementia Unit at a long-term care facility in Brooklyn, New York. Mr. George's next of kin is his daughter, Sharon Pryce. His medical diagnosis included advanced dementia, hypertension, type 2 diabetes, and hypercholesterolemia. Mr. George required one person to assist him with all his activities of daily living (ADLs), except bed mobility and transfer in and out of bed. With these tasks he required two persons to assist him. He uses a wheelchair as his mode of mobility and needs to be wheeled. He is incontinent of bowel and bladder. He is able to feed himself after his meal trays are set up, but requires encouragement or assistance to complete his meals.

Two months after Mr. George was admitted to the facility as a resident, he was observed to have a pressure ulcer in his mid-sacrum. The wound-care team was called to assess the ulcer and make clinical decisions as necessary. The multidisciplinary team included the wound-care nurse, unit physician, unit nurse, nursing supervisor, dietitian, and occupational therapist. On assessment by the wound-care nurse, the ulcer bed was covered with approximately 75% yellowish tissue called slough and 25% pink tissue. The ulcer was identified as a stage 3 pressure ulcer. The physician ordered immediate treatment for Mr. George, and pressure-relieving devices were put in place. The dietitian evaluated Mr. George's recent blood test results and recommended supplements that would aid in the healing of the ulcer. Sharon, his daughter, was notified of the ulcer development.

Background

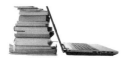

Sharon was unable to provide for her father's needs due to his advancing medical diagnosis of dementia. Sharon wanted to select a facility for her father located in a neighborhood close to where she lived in Brooklyn, and decided to use the website Nursing Home Compare to help her evaluate potential long-term care facilities. The website gave the nursing home she selected a five-star rating, which made her feel comfortable with her decision to admit her father there.

The Nursing Home Compare website is an official U.S. government site for Medicare (www.medicare.gov/nhcompare). The website provides detailed information on all Medicare- and Medicaid-certified nursing homes in the country. It compares the quality of nursing homes, using a five-star rating system based on health inspection results, nursing-home staff data, quality measures, and fire safety inspection results.

The standard protocol for a long-term care facility is that all residents should have a complete assessment, which includes a body assessment by a nurse and a physician upon admission. After investigation, one nurse recalled that Mr. George's sacral area was purplish in color when he was admitted, but there was no documentation in his files to corroborate this assertion. A purple discoloration on a pressure site can be evident of a deep tissue injury, which indicates that there is injury to the underlying soft tissue due to pressure.

Next Steps

Sharon is scheduled to meet with the administrator of the facility to discuss the development of her father's stage 3 ulcer. Sharon would like an answer as to why her father developed this ulcer after only two months in the facility. Sharon plans to bring her lawyer to the meeting. Prior to the meeting, the administrator will consult with the wound-care team to better understand Mr. George's condition and the circumstances behind the development of the pressure ulcer.

Discussion Questions

1. As the administrator, how would you respond to this situation?

2. How should the administrator work with the wound-care team in developing a response?

3. Who do you think bears the primary responsibility in the development of the pressure ulcer?

4. Do you think the Nursing Home Compare website was an effective tool for Sharon?

5. What programs should the administrator consider implementing to avoid the development of pressure ulcers in high-risk residents?

Case 57

CASE CONTRIBUTOR **James A. Johnson**

Situation

Joan is an 86-year-old woman who came to Colly County Memorial Hospital with dyspnea, fever, chills, and a persistent cough.[1] She was diagnosed as having pneumonia, underlying conditions of malnutrition, and Alzheimer's disease. She was admitted into the hospital for medical management.

At the time of her arrival, the hospital was filled to capacity, but a bed would be available within an hour as a discharge was in process on the medical/surgical unit. Admitting orders were initiated in the emergency room, and Joan was taken to the radiology department for a chest x-ray while waiting for a room. The radiology department was busy and operating with less than full staff because three workers were out sick. It was 2 o'clock, and no staff had been able to eat lunch.

A registered technician, Pamela, wheeled Joan to one of the x-ray rooms, closed the door, and proceeded to lift Joan from her wheelchair and hoist her onto the examination table. Pamela knew that she was breaking the hospital policy requiring two technicians per patient. Pamela was an experienced technician and had worked at the hospital for several years. After the x-ray, Pamela assisted Joan from the examination table to the wheelchair, but during the transfer, Joan lost her balance and fell to the floor. Joan complained of a slight hip pain while Pamela was helping her up, but Pamela decided not to write an incident report. Although concerned, Pamela was afraid of the repercussions of reporting the incident. She hoped that Joan would become confused about the fall and forget about it. She then made arrangements for Joan to be taken to her room.

Two hours later, Joan's daughter notified the nurse that Joan had told her about the fall and the pain in her hip. The daughter demanded to know when the fall had occurred and why she had not been notified. Joan underwent a hip examination that showed a fracture had resulted from the fall.

Next Steps

When confronted, Pamela denied any knowledge of the incident. Concerned by the allegation, hospital administration conducted a thorough review. Further investigation into Pamela's background revealed that she had been terminated from her previous job because of a similar incident. However, Pamela had recorded a different reason on her job application at Colly County Memorial Hospital.

Discussion Questions

1. If you were Pamela's supervisor, which issues would you address?

2. What are the possible outcomes of this incident for (a) you as the supervisor, (b) Pamela, (c) the radiology department, and (d) the hospital?

3. As the hospital administrator, what policies could you enact to improve the quality of your hiring decisions?

4. If Pamela reported the incident to you as her supervisor, what process would you need to follow?

Reference

[1] Kilpatrick, A. O., & Johnson, J. A. (1999). *Human resources and organizational behavior: Cases in health services management.* Chicago, IL: Health Administration Press.

Case 58

HIV Testing at a Health and Fitness Fair

CASE CONTRIBUTOR **Sharon Williams Lewis**

Situation

An annual health and fitness fair was being held at a convention center in an urban metropolitan city. As in previous years, thousands of people were expected to attend. Activities offered to participants included free health tests and screenings, health education, nutrition, and fitness demonstrations. Because of the high incidence of HIV in this urban city, screening tests for HIV were featured in the print and news media advertisements for the health fair. Dr. Susan Jones, the branch manager of laboratory services of the local Department of Health, was responsible for overseeing community laboratory testing. Dr. Jones assigned Mark Taylor, medical technologist, to monitor and conduct observations of all booths that were providing laboratory testing and screens at the health fair. The Herman Health Group was the only registered vendor administering the rapid HIV test of all the laboratory screening groups.

While setting up the booth for HIV testing, the representative did not conduct the quality control testing for the new lot of test kits brought to the health fair. The quality control testing includes use of reagents designated for negative and positive readings that are used to check the performance or accuracy of the test kit. Additionally, there was no method to assure that the temperature storage of the test kits was maintained in accordance with the manufacturer's recommendations. The location of the booth did not provide client privacy for testing, consultation of test results, or education on HIV. It was quickly determined that the representative from the Herman Health Group would require close supervision.

Mr. Taylor conducted observations of the Herman Health Group's booth. The group's operator explained the testing procedure to a client. The client swabbed with the kit's flat pad the outer gum both upper and lower as instructed. Next the flat pad was placed in the testing device. The client was then informed it would take 20 minutes before the test result could be read based on the manufacturer's instructions. In response, the client informed the operator after 15 minutes that he could not wait any longer. Complying with the client's request, the operator checked the device for a result. The client was given literature and informed the HIV screen result was negative. The supervisor for the operator and owner of the Herman Health Group arrived mid-day to see how things were going. The Herman Health Group is registered with the local Department of Health to perform community HIV screening tests among other outreach program activities. Mr. Taylor interviewed the supervisor and asked about training requirements of the staff who conduct the tests. Although the supervisor stated extensive training had been provided, there was no evidence that staff competency was checked prior to the field assignments. As a result of Herman Health

Group's failure to follow manufacturer's instructions when administering a rapid HIV test, the booth was closed by the Department of Health.

Background

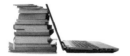

HIV is a retrovirus that infects the cells of the immune system destroying or impairing their function. HIV can progress to acquired immune deficiency syndrome (AIDS). Early detection and treatment intervention can prevent or delay the progression of HIV to AIDS. The Joint United Nations Programme on HIV (UNAIDS) and the U.S. Centers for Disease Control and Prevention (CDC) define high prevalence of HIV/AIDS at greater than 1%.[1] Interestingly, the District of Columbia reported an overall prevalence of 3.2% for persons living with HIV/AIDS and 7.6% prevalence among 40- to 49-year-olds in its 2010 annual report.[2] The World Health Organization indicates people between the ages of 40 and 49 are most affected with HIV. According to the Kaiser Family Foundation, prevalence of HIV/AIDS for the same age group worldwide was 0.8% in 2010 and 0.6% for the United States in 2009, the most recent year available.[3]

Nationally, there has been an increase in news and print media on the importance of knowing your HIV status and providing education on prevention. Many Departments of Health, local governments, and health organizations have developed educational materials for dissemination and news media campaigns on HIV prevention. In addition, health professionals have provided training on how to perform testing with HIV screening test kits approved by the Food and Drug Administration (FDA) in anticipation of reaching a wider segment of the population. Clients who have a positive result from the HIV screening test are informed to go for a confirmatory serum test. The integrity of the proficiency in using proper technique when conducting screening tests is as important for poorly performed false negative results as it is for accurate positive results.

Next Steps

The large number of participants attending the health and fitness fair's annual event was an excellent opportunity for educational outreach on HIV/AIDS and screening. Administration of HIV screening tests in accordance with the manufacturer's recommendations is imperative for accurate results. As the monitor for the Department of Health, Mr. Taylor faced a number of competing issues that required decisions. At one extreme was shutting down the Herman Health Group's booth given the failure of the operator to use proper testing procedures. There was always a middle-ground option to keep the booth open for face-to-face interactions and dissemination of educational materials, as well as referrals to other test sites. On the other hand, the more challenging dilemma was what to do, if anything, with those clients who had already been tested by the Herman Health Group and may have received inaccurate results. By not contacting these clients, would Mr. Taylor be putting them, and others, at risk?

Discussion Questions

1. Is it appropriate for Mr. Taylor and the Department of Health to suspend all testing by the Herman Health Group?

2. Should previously tested clients be contacted and retested? If yes, discuss how to implement the notification process?

3. What is the responsibility of Herman Health Group's supervisor in this scenario? As the supervisor, how would you handle this situation?

4. What impact, if any, would the reported test results from the Herman Health Group have on the local prevalence rates?

References

[1] World Health Organization. (2012). *Health topics, HIV/AIDS*. Retrieved from http://www.who.int/topics/hiv_aids/en/

[2] District of Columbia, Department of Health HIV/AIDS, Hepatitis, STD, and TB Administration. (2010). *HIV/AIDS, hepatitis, STD, and TB administration annual report 2010*. Retrieved from http://www.dchealth.dc.gov/doh/frames.asp?doc=/doh/lib/doh/services/administration_offices/hiv_aids/pdf/2010_Annual_Report_FINAL.pdf

[3] Kaiser Family Foundation. (2010). *United States global health policy, adult HIV/AIDS prevalence rate (Aged 15–49)*. Retrieved from http://www.globalhealthfacts.org/data/topic/map.aspx?ind=3

Case 59

To Hear This Message in Korean, Press 9

CASE CONTRIBUTOR Scott D. Musch

Situation

Angela, the program coordinator for a federally qualified health center (FQHC) in Queens, New York, was concerned that the language and cultural capabilities of the staff at the health center were not keeping pace with the diverse community. The FQHC, one of several in the Queens Borough, is located in a designated Medically Underserved Area (MUA) neighborhood and assists underserved populations, homeless people, and migrant workers. MUAs are areas designated by the federal government as having too few primary care providers, high infant mortality, high poverty, and/or high elderly population. Most of the health center patients are at incomes below the poverty level and nearly two-thirds are racial or ethnic minorities. The mission of the health center is to be community based and patient focused, which can be a challenge given the cross-cultural and language differences.

Immigrant populations have swelled around the health center over the last decade. The clinic's staff is increasingly confronting language and cultural challenges. Almost daily, Angela shares in the frustrations of practitioners trying to best serve their patients in spite of these barriers. Most immigrants can speak enough English to get around in their daily activities, but that skill level is usually insufficient in the doctor's office when discussing medical terms. Miscommunication or lack of communication due to cultural sensitivities can lead to ineffective patient care, including errors in diagnoses, mistranslations, and misunderstandings in treatment instructions. These language and cultural challenges may even discourage people from seeking health care at the center. Angela recognizes that the center may not be fully realizing its mission to serve the community.

Much of the staff at the center is bilingual, but they predominantly speak only Spanish and English. This has served the clinic generally well as the largest demographic group aside from Whites is Hispanic or Latino minorities (see Table 59–1). However, as the community has become more diverse, there is a need for other languages and cultural skills, particularly to serve Asian communities. The existing interpretation services at the health center are largely insufficient to deal with this evolving problem. The majority of residents in the community speak a language other than English at home (see Table 59–2). However, the health center is inadequately prepared to handle multiple languages. The operator service on the phone, for instance, provides language services only in English or Spanish. Angela wonders how many potential patients hang up when trying to schedule an appointment at the center due to frustration of not being able to understand enough to get through the menus. The management team recognizes the increasing need to recruit more multilingual staff and hire interpreters. The health center has hired interpreter services, but they can cost up to $190 an hour, which can be very expensive for a nonprofit organization.

Table 59–1 Selected Demographics: Queens County, New York

Race	Percentage of Population
White (alone)	30.2%
Hispanic or Latino (of any race)	26.9%
Puerto Rican	5.3%
Mexican	3.6%
Other	18.0%
Asian (alone)	21.9%
Chinese	8.5%
Asian Indian	6.0%
Korean	2.6%
Filipino	2.0%
Japanese	0.2%
Other	2.6%
Black or African American (alone)	17.6%
American Indian and Alaska Native (alone)	0.3%
Other race (alone)	1.6%
Two or more races	1.5%

Source: *Queens County, New York, ACS Demographic and Housing Estimates: 2009, American Community Survey*, U.S. Census Bureau.[1]

Table 59–2 Selected Demographics: Queens County, New York

Language Spoken at Home (Population 5 years and over)	Percentage of Population
English only	44.2%
Language other than English	55.8%
Speak English less than "very well"	28.5%
Spanish	23.8%
Speak English less than "very well"	12.6%
Other Indo-European languages	16.8%
Speak English less than "very well"	7.2%
Asian and Pacific Islander languages	13.5%
Speak English less than "very well"	8.1%
Other languages	1.7%

Source: *Queens County, New York, Selected Social Characteristics in the United States: 2009, American Community Survey*, U.S. Census Bureau.[2]

Background

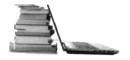

The demographics of the U.S. population over the next 40 years will experience significant changes. The Pew Research Center estimates that 82% of the increase in the U.S. population (117 million) will be attributed to new immigrants (67 million) arriving from 2005 to 2050 and their U.S.-born descendents (50 million).[3] The report states that by 2050 nearly one in five Americans (19%) will be an immigrant. According to the U.S. Census Bureau's American Community Survey, the percent of people who are foreign born in New York State is 21.3%, which is above the national average of 12.4%, and within Queens County in New York, the percent is more than double at 46.6%.[4]

The demographic trends in the U.S. population highlight the need for more diversity among healthcare professions. Greater diversity will lead to improved public health by providing patients with increased opportunities to see practitioners who share their common race, language, ethnicity, and culture. In its study "The Rationale for Diversity in the Health Professions: A Review of the Evidence," the Health Resources and Services Administration found compelling evidence to support a diverse health professions workforce:

- "minority patients tend to receive better interpersonal care from practitioners of their own race or ethnicity, particularly in primary care and mental health settings;
- non-English-speaking patients experience better interpersonal care, greater medical comprehension, and greater likelihood of keeping follow-up appointments when they see a language-concordant practitioner, particularly in mental health care."[5]

Next Steps

Angela recognizes that there are tremendous needs in the immigrant communities in Queens County that are not being met. While the health center provides quality care, there needs to be a mechanism in place to deal with language and cultural barriers to improve interactions between patients and health professionals.

Discussion Questions

1. How should Angela and the management team address this challenge?

2. Do patients have a fundamental right to an interpreter?

3. Should the staff of a community health center and FQHC reflect the diversity of the population they serve?

4. If so, what are some of the challenges an organization will face trying to realize that objective?

References

[1] U.S. Census Bureau. (n.d.). Queens County, New York, ACS Demographic and Housing Estimates: 2009, American Community Survey. Retrieved from http://factfinder.census.gov/servlet/ADPTable?_bm=y&-geo_id=05000US36081&-qr_name=ACS_2009_1YR_G00_DP5&-context=adp&-ds_name=&-tree_id=309&-_lang=en&-redoLog=false&-format=

[2] U.S. Census Bureau. (n.d.). Queens County, New York, Selected Social Characteristics in the United States; 2009, American Community Survey. Retrieved from http://factfinder.census.gov/

servlet/ADPTable?_bm=y&-geo_id=05000US36081&-qr_name=ACS_2009_1YR_G00_
DP2&-context=adp&-ds_name=&-tree_id=309&-_lang=en&-redoLog=false&-format=

[3] Passel, J. S., & Cohn, D. (2008, February 11). *U.S. population projections: 2005–2050.*
Pew Research Center Report. Retrieved from http://pewhispanic.org/files/reports/85.pdf

[4] U.S. Census Bureau. (n.d.). 2005–2009 American Community Survey 5-Year Estimates. Retrieved
from http://factfinder.census.gov/servlet/GCTTable?_bm=y&-geo_id=01000US&-_box_head_
nbr=GCT0501&-ds_name=ACS_2009_5YR_G00_&-_lang=en&-mt_name=ACS_2009_
5YR_G00_GCT0501_US9F&-format=US-9F

[5] U.S. Department of Health and Human Services, Health Resources and Services Administration,
Bureau of Health Professions. (2006, October). The rationale for diversity in the health professions:
A review of the evidence. Retrieved from ftp://ftp.hrsa.gov/bhpr/workforce/diversity.pdf

Case 60

Blackout 2003—An Environmental Health Response

CASE CONTRIBUTOR **Anthony Drautz**

Situation

The post 9/11 era and the influx of natural and manmade disasters worldwide in the last decade have heightened the awareness of the limited resources many public health agencies have in dealing with emergencies and the first response capabilities of local public health agencies. In August 2003, many parts of the Northeast and Midwest regions in the United States and parts of Ontario, Canada, experienced a blackout caused by the malfunction of the electrical power grid that supplies electric power. It is suspected this malfunction was a result of a tree branch that was neglected and fell on a power line, triggering a domino effect that eliminated power affecting tens of millions of users creating among other things a concern for public health officials.

The incident occurred during a week in which classic motor vehicle enthusiasts invade southeast Michigan culminating in a one-day event known as the Woodward Dream Cruise. This event attracts what has been estimated at over one million cruisers and fans of classic vehicles. Jane, a local health department's Environmental Health Administrator, knew that she would need to rely on the cooperation and expertise of not only her staff but other partner agencies in the region. With no water, no power, no sanitary facilities, a potentially compromised food supply, and temperatures in the mid 90s, the potential for a public health disaster was a real possibility and it was "back to basics" from a public health management perspective.

Background

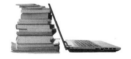

While the Woodward Dream Cruise is hosted primarily in one of the three largest counties that comprise the Detroit, Michigan metropolitan area, the magnitude of the event and the ensuing disaster affected the entire region. State and local agencies responding to the disaster all had unique interests to consider when responding to the incident and circulating information to the public. Providing a clear, consistent message proved to be a challenge for Jane and other local administrators. From the time it takes to boil water to avoid a waterborne illness, to the enforcement of safe food regulations to avoid foodborne illness outbreaks, each local public health department and state department involved in the response disseminated information that varied from agency to agency.

Jane realized quickly that the immediate restoration of basic needs of the general population affected by a natural or manmade disaster is related to the rapid response and accessibility of the environmental health workforce. Her environmental health workforce has a shared responsibility for the monitoring, evaluation, and education of the population to reestablish access to or provide resources to obtain safe drinking water and food and restore sanitation protections to prevent disease transmission. Environmental health expertise is relied upon in these events and can prevent the occurrence and spread of numerous communicable diseases that may lead to widespread epidemics. Emergency and contingency planning and the ability to deploy competent environmental health professionals are keys to preparation for disaster response. Contradicting messages between agencies regarding the safe sanitation practices can frustrate and exacerbate the problem for an anxious public. Jane was well aware of the sensitivity and importance of disseminating information to the public.

Response and assistance to populations affected by natural disasters begin and end at the local level. Federal and state monetary aid, support staff, and material resources are often delayed and are not sustained after the initial response efforts conclude. It is critical that local environmental health agencies are proactive in their commitment to ongoing planning and staffing competent personnel to address the challenges of natural and manmade disasters. Recent hurricanes, tsunamis, earthquakes, and floods have identified gaps in the capabilities of the environmental health workforce to respond to these catastrophic events. Multiple events in a relatively short period of time further strain the availability of essential personnel to respond to natural and manmade disasters in adequate numbers to address the immediate needs of the affected population. These considerations are most important for agencies at high levels in the organization during the strategic planning process, but often are not included.

Next Steps

In the event of widespread or multiple disaster events, aid, support, and resources will be strained and the multijurisdictional or unified incident command structure will be critical in a successful disaster-related response. Additional problems will ensue if careful, structured, and proactive emergency public health planning strategies are not met. Jane and her staff worked to ensure public health staffing needs were addressed before they became necessitated. Demands on an already depleted public health workforce could exacerbate existing tribulations as staff were deployed or reassigned and fatigued by ongoing, multiple, and perpetual efforts. Caution and recognition of these obstacles were considered by Jane when planning for disaster relief staffing. Burnout and fatigue often accompany extended deployment of staff to horrendous, unsanitary settings. Consequently, the ability of her staff to perform assigned duties will lessen.

In addition to environmental health staff, physicians, nurses, epidemiologists, mental health professionals, and health educators must be familiar with the Incident Command System and be trained and available as appropriate, to deploy to such disasters. Environmental health support is often complicated by obstacles that involve the other public health disciplines. Special needs victims have been identified as a challenge when responding to public health emergencies. Physical and mental handicaps, overcrowding of relief centers, improper sanitary practices, and security issues are all examples of problems that can be addressed by a multidisciplinary response approach. Traditional first responders (police, fire, EMS) must have an increased awareness of the role of public health in situational emergency response. These partnerships should be created and maintained by Jane prior to an event.

In relation to safe drinking water and food, relief efforts may be delayed, which further adds to the frustration of first responder emergency relief workers. It is imperative that immediate survival techniques are mastered and can be effectively communicated to masses of the population in an affected area. This includes personnel of other agencies that may partner in response and relief efforts.

Environmental health successes following a natural or manmade disaster can be attributed to building and maintaining partnerships and workforce development prior to the event. Partnerships should include public, private, volunteer, and charitable organizations. Private sector inclusion is a viable approach in assisting with response and relief efforts. Intergovernmental agreements or memorandums of understanding should be secured with local, state, and federal agencies. Volunteer and charitable organizational resource commitments should also be arranged to provide additional support. Jane must be cognizant that due to the unpredictable nature and magnitude of natural or manmade disasters collaborative efforts will ensure that adequate personnel deployments are made to assist in the restoration of basic needs of affected victims.

Environmental health workforce development and partnership efforts continue to improve. Jane's staff is no exception. The Centers for Disease Control and Prevention have developed a framework for building the capacity of the 10 essential services of environmental health (see Table 60–1).[1]

In order to facilitate a rapid, effective, efficient, and comprehensive environmental health response to victims of natural or manmade disasters, continuous emergency preparedness planning and workforce development of Jane and her staff is crucial.

Table 60–1 10 Essential Environmental Public Health Services

1. **Monitor** environmental and health status to identify and solve community environmental health problems
2. **Diagnose and investigate** environmental health problems and health hazards in the community
3. **Inform, educate, and empower** people about environmental health issues
4. **Mobilize** community partnerships and actions to identify and solve environmental health problems
5. **Develop policies and plans** that support individual and community environmental health efforts
6. **Enforce** laws and regulations that protect environmental health and ensure safety
7. **Link** people to needed environmental health services and assure the provision of environmental health services when otherwise unavailable
8. **Assure** a competent environmental health workforce
9. **Evaluate** effectiveness, accessibility, and quality of personal and population-based environmental health services
10. **Research** for new insights and innovative solutions to environmental health problems and issues

Source: "10 Essential Environmental Public Health Services," National Center for Environmental Health, Centers for Disease Control and Prevention, 2010.

Discussion Questions

1. What are the tools necessary for Jane to effectively manage a public health emergency?

2. How does the flexibility of Jane's environmental health workforce strengthen the capabilities of the public health response to an incident?

3. Do public health officials have a role in the emergency response to natural and manmade disasters?

4. Do the media assist or hinder response efforts? Explain.

Reference

[1] National Center for Environmental Health. (2010, January 25). *10 Essential Environmental Public Health Services*. Retrieved from Centers for Disease Control and Prevention at http://www.cdc.gov/nceh/ehs/Home/HealthService.htm

Case 61

Communicating the Need for Hospital Consolidation

CASE CONTRIBUTOR **David Meckstroth**

Situation

Returning to his office after a meeting, Steve receives another fax listing many questions from one of the local newspapers pertaining to the potential consolidation of two hospitals in West Central Ohio. Steve, the new president and chief executive officer (CEO) of Upper Valley Medical Center, has been dealing with organized opposition from a group called Save Our Hospitals (SOH), numerous questions from newspapers, and has been caught in a communication whirlwind involving the consolidation.

There had been discussions for several years about the possibility of a major acute care consolidation, long before the previous CEO left to pursue another opportunity. Through multiple strategic planning sessions and feasibility studies prepared by Ernst & Young, the future strategic direction for Upper Valley Medical Center was being critically evaluated. Upper Valley Medical Center is the nonprofit parent corporation that owned two acute care hospitals, one behavioral science hospital, three long-term care facilities, a for-profit insurance company, 11 medical office buildings, a home health agency, one free-standing dialysis center, and a corporation that employed physicians. All of these entities are in Miami County, located in West Central Ohio.

The population of Miami County was approximately 110,000 and the two acute care hospitals were located in the cities of Piqua and Troy. Both cities had a population of nearly 22,000, and they were the largest cities in the county. Piqua is located more to the north of the county and Troy located more to the south. The two hospitals served different markets. However, there was some competition in the north market and major competition in the south market, causing additional pressures on the hospitals.

Hospital management and Ernst & Young considered all feasible alternatives with the final decision to construct a new hospital in the middle of the county. Of the possible alternatives, the new hospital provided the best long-term financial viability option. The consolidation of acute care services to one location was estimated to save more than $15 million annually in operating expenses. After thoroughly evaluating the possible alternatives, Steve believed the health system would not be viable in the long-term without the new hospital.

The location would be five miles south of Piqua and five miles north of Troy. Upper Valley Medical Center owned approximately 140 acres of land at the new site. At one time, there had been an acute care hospital at this location, but the acute care services had been discontinued and transferred to the hospitals in Piqua and Troy. The former acute care hospital was converted to business and administrative offices.

The formal announcement of a new hospital led to a large public outcry as to why Upper Valley Medical Center would want to close two apparently well-run hospitals and build a new facility in the middle of the county. City officials in Piqua and Troy had significant concerns over the plan. SOH opened two storefronts in Piqua and Troy to distribute information, most of which was inaccurate.

To gain strength, SOH incorporated and sought funding through contributions. The primary funding source, however, came from a retired primary care physician who had a large following from his many patients and families he had served during his career. In addition, he was the current Miami County Coroner and was well known. His family had contributed significant dollars in previous years to the hospital in Troy.

SOH created large signs and bright red bumper stickers that attracted much attention. The leadership of SOH contacted the State of Ohio Attorney General's Office on a weekly basis in an attempt to get her to intervene and stop the plans for a new hospital. In addition, SOH contacted the local newspapers frequently to gain publicity. The two local newspapers, *Piqua Daily Call* and *Troy Daily News*, and one regional paper, *Dayton Daily News*, covered the story almost daily. Reporters at the papers routinely faxed multiple questions to the communications department at Upper Valley Medical Center.

Steve had multiple organizational constituents to consider in how he handled communications. Each constituent seemed to have an opinion of what should be communicated and how it should be delivered. In order to assist in handling the multiple communication issues, Steve formed a board of director's Communication Committee. The members of the committee included Steve, the director of communications, and three trustees from the board of directors. The Communication's Committee was authorized by the board of directors to provide oversight of communications, which helped to streamline the communication process.

The primary constituents included 21 board of directors, 50 foundation board members, 250 medical staff members, 200 volunteers, 2000 employees, thousands of patients, and the general public. Before long, Steve was consumed in public relation issues and was spending nearly 50% of his time on communications. Most, if not all, responses became part of the public record, which added further complications in the certificate of need (CON) process. Moreover, SOH filed a lawsuit with the Miami County Common Pleas Court in an attempt to obtain a temporary and permanent injunction and a declaratory judgment against Upper Valley Medical Center in order to prevent it from moving forward with the plan to build a new hospital.

Background

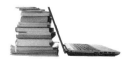

In order to construct a new hospital, Upper Valley Medical Center was required by the State of Ohio to obtain approval of a CON. States require CONs in order to optimize the use of healthcare resources. Hospitals subject to CON requirements must demonstrate a tangible healthcare need or other compelling justification in order to receive approval. A community's input and desires also affect the outcome of CON requests.

As the CON process unfolded, there were multiple public hearings. Each hearing was fairly contentious with many SOH members attending. The entity that was required to conduct the hearings and make a recommendation to the State of Ohio was the Miami Valley Health Improvement Council (MVHIC). The CON law in Ohio had been changed a year earlier and essentially a positive recommendation from the MVHIC would result in the CON being approved by the director of health for the State of Ohio. If the MVHIC recommended denial of the CON, the director of health could still approve the CON although this would be very unlikely.

There were many questions as to the financial feasibility of building a new hospital. SOH expressed their support for the existing hospitals and saw no reason to build a new facility. Steve had facilitated evaluating the feasibility of maintaining both hospitals, closing either the hospital in Piqua or Troy and consolidating all operations to the other facility, or constructing a new hospital while closing the existing two facilities. The feasibility studies were very clear that the only likely viable long-term option was to build a new hospital. The primary reason was the belief that significant market share would be lost if one hospital was simply closed and operations were consolidated in the remaining hospital.

Upper Valley Medical Center found itself on the front page of both local papers virtually every day along with being the subject of multiple letters to the editor. All of the articles and letters were reviewed by the MVHIC as being relevant to the CON process. In fact, the MVHIC encouraged individuals to express their opinion. Many concerns were expressed about the additional distance people and ambulances would have to travel to a new facility. SOH members voiced concern that the additional distance would cost lives since it would take longer to get to the new hospital in emergency situations. In addition, adding to the public discourse was the fact that the new hospital location was not within either municipality. Piqua and Troy would lose significant local income tax revenue, though some income tax revenue would flow back to the residences of the hospital employees.

Despite the public opposition, Upper Valley Medical Center had many supporters. Approximately 90% of practicing physicians supported the direction toward a new hospital and signed a petition indicating their support. Many individuals in the community wrote letters of support. However, SOH members were confrontational and boisterous, which resulted in many supporters preferring to keep a low profile. Many Upper Valley Medical Center employees removed their identification badges when in public for fear of being accosted by an SOH member.

Typically in the CON process, the MVHIC would host the final hearing near the organization requesting a CON. Due to the public controversy throughout this process, however, MVHIC decided to move the final hearing to Miami Valley Hospital in Dayton, approximately 35 miles away from Miami County. SOH chartered three large buses to bring nearly 200 members to attend the final hearing. Majority approval of the 22 MVHIC board members would be required to grant the CON.

Next Steps

Steve realized that his success in handling the external, as well as the internal, communication challenges would greatly affect whether Upper Valley Medical Center obtained CON approval. Without approval, the future viability of the health system was in jeopardy. However, even with approval, the protests from SOH were not likely to go away anytime soon. SOH would clearly remain an adversarial constituent that would need to be addressed.

Steve evaluated the optimal communication strategy for Upper Valley Medical Center. His approach had to be proactive as there was significant erroneous information being circulated by SOH. Steve recognized the importance of displaying confidence to the organization's constituents and doing his best to dispel their concerns. However, he also recognized the challenge of needing to address each fax of questions he received daily from the local newspapers. Each question, no matter how insignificant it might appear, required a decision. Should we respond? If so, how should we respond? Who should be involved in crafting a response? Who should be informed of the response? It seemed like an endless cycle.

Discussion Questions

1. How do you think Steve should coordinate communications in his role? Should there be different communication approaches for internal versus external constituencies? Should there be a different approach if Upper Valley Medical Center was a for-profit entity?

2. Recognizing that all responses would likely become public information, how would this affect your approach?

3. How would you manage communications in this scenario given the large number of stakeholders with various levels of knowledge and needs?

4. Recognizing that to effectively address the communication issues would be very time-consuming, what if any organizational structure changes would you implement to enable you to have sufficient time?

5. Knowing how emotional and volatile the situation is, as CEO how much of your time would you dedicate to handling the communications? Would believing that the new hospital is imperative to the long-term financial viability of the system affect your approach?

6. If Upper Valley Medical Center receives CON approval, what should it do in the coming months/years to garner support recognizing that SOH members will likely never support the new hospital?

Case 62 | A *Giardia* Outbreak?

CASE CONTRIBUTOR Scott D. Musch

Situation

"This is the tenth confirmed case of giardiasis we received this week," relayed Eric, to one of the department's environmental engineers. Eric works as an environmental health specialist in the Northwest Region office of the Pennsylvania Department of Environmental Protection (DEP), Bureau of Water Standards and Facility Regulation. Several physicians in the local township called his office this week to report positive laboratory tests of *Giardia* cysts in their patients, who were experiencing flu-like illnesses with symptoms of persistent diarrhea, nausea, and abdominal cramps. The physicians were growing concerned of a potential outbreak of a waterborne contaminant in the community's water supply, yet they hadn't seen any public announcements from the DEP. Officials from the local health department had also called earlier in the day to ask if any boil water advisories should be in effect.

One of Eric's essential duties in his job as an environmental health specialist is to respond to and investigate complaints and violations of Pennsylvania's water supply and wastewater treatment facilities. His department develops surveillance strategies that direct field inspector activities at water supply and wastewater treatment facilities. In addition, he works closely with the Bureau of Watershed Management, which is responsible for planning and managing the water resources in Pennsylvania, including monitoring and regulating water sources to ensure safe drinking water, as required by the Safe Drinking Water Act (SDWA).

The local township is a small city in rural Pennsylvania with a population of less than 8000 located near the Allegheny National Forest. Eric knows that many rural cities in the mountainous areas of Pennsylvania are particularly susceptible to waterborne contaminants since their water supplies from lakes, ponds, or streams can become contaminated with animal droppings or human sewage discharge. Although water treatment plants have been constructed in many communities, some of the more remote areas still did not have completely effective water systems that were fully risk compliant. Eric remembered studying the *Giardia* outbreak that occurred in 1979 in Bradford City, a community not too dissimilar to the local township.

Background

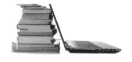

Giardia and *Cryptosporidium* are the most common etiologic agents causing waterborne outbreaks in the United States. *Giardia* and *Cryptosporidium* are protozoan intestinal parasites that cause diarrheal illnesses in people. The parasites are found in every region of the United States and throughout the world. The cysts of the organisms are commonly transmitted from the environment to humans through contaminated water or food. The illnesses associated with the parasites, giardiasis and cryptosporidiosis, are usually acute and can become chronic and last up to one or two months. From 1965 to 1996, there were 118 outbreaks of giardiasis in the United States with 26,305 reported cases of illness, mainly attributed to the consumption of contaminated drinking water from public and individual water systems with the majority of cases occurring due to inadequately treated surface water systems.[1]

The state of Pennsylvania was once among the leaders nationally in the number of recorded waterborne disease outbreaks.[2] The *Giardia* outbreak in Bradford City in 1979 is an informative reference case. Bradford's water system is supplied from three upland reservoirs. A reservoir is an artificial lake created in a river valley by a dam or built by excavation to store water. Prior to the outbreak, the water from the reservoirs was delivered directly to consumers without any filtration or other barriers. Treatment relied exclusively on chlorination. The water passed out of the reservoirs into the transmission mains. During September to December 1979, 3500 cases of giardiasis occurred in Bradford.[3] A number of events led to this outbreak. First, even though chlorination treatment was provided, it was interrupted and deficient at times. Second, heavy rains caused runoff in the watershed leading to high turbidity. Turbidity is a key test of water quality and represents the cloudiness in water caused by suspended particles. Incidentally, Bradford had applied for and was granted a waiver from the U.S. Environmental Protection Agency of its obligation to notify the public of the high turbidity measures in the water supply. Although chlorinated, the water was unfiltered prior to passing through the transmission mains. Third, beavers in the watershed were infected with *Giardia* cysts contributing to the infection of the water supply. In order to ensure that no future outbreaks of the disease occurred, Bradford City constructed a water treatment plant to treat all water delivered to the city. The facility was capable of removing all microorganisms from the water through chemical treatment and filtration.

Next Steps

Eric's department had been in the process of evaluating local monitoring and sampling equipment in the area, so the field inspection surveys for the local township might have been delayed. If this turned out to be the beginning of an outbreak, his department could be in store for some harsh criticism. The environmental engineers were in the process of coordinating with local inspectors to collect more data, and Eric thought that this may be the best course of action before alerting the public of a waterborne disease outbreak. Eric sat down, and reflected on the best course of action to take. He considered calling the local health officials to update them on the situation. Eric thought it might be prudent to ask the local media to alert residents to boil water before consumption. However, his department still needed to determine the cause and he didn't want to risk alarming the public unnecessarily. He knew he should coordinate any external communication activity first with his supervisor, even if it delayed getting the message out to the public. He picked up the phone to call his supervisor and ask for recommendations.

Discussion Questions

1. What course of action should Eric follow if inspection tests confirm that the local township's water supply is contaminated by *Giardia*?

2. What parties should Eric involve in the process of determining an appropriate response by the department?

3. Should Eric release an official boil water notice to inform the public as a precaution? What factors should Eric consider to determine the optimal time?

References

[1] United States Environmental Protection Agency, Office of Water. (1998, August). Giardia: Human health criteria document (EPA No. 823R002). Retrieved from http://water.epa.gov/action/advisories/drinking/upload/2009_02_03_criteria_humanhealth_microbial_giardia.pdf

[2] Pennsylvania Department of Environmental Protection, Bureau of Water Standards and Facility Regulation. (2009, November). Cryptosporidium and Giardia . . . Are they in YOUR drinking water? (3800-BK-DEP0524). Retrieved from http://www.elibrary.dep.state.pa.us/dsweb/Get/Document-77461/3800-BK-DEP0524.pdf

[3] Karanis, P., Kourenti, C., & Smith, H. (2007). Waterborne transmission of protozoan parasites: A worldwide review of outbreaks and lessons learnt. *Journal of Water and Health, 5*(1), 1–38. doi: 10.2166/wh.2006.002

Case 63

Senior Cyber Café

CASE CONTRIBUTOR Scott D. Musch

Situation

Linda, president of the Mid Florida Area Agency on Aging in Gainesville, was concerned about complaints she had received from several seniors at the local senior center. The complaints involved two of her volunteers, Kim and Mark, college students from a local technical school. Kim and Mark were new volunteers at the agency and, given their computer proficiency, they were greatly needed. They had explained to Linda that they were volunteering in order to "give back to the community," but probably also to augment their resumes. Linda put their computer skills to great use and asked them to teach computer-training classes two times a week at the local senior center as part of a Senior Cyber Café program. The program was a new initiative for the agency and Linda had great expectations. The program consisted of a 10-week computer training class that provided instruction on basic computer use including how to access the Internet and use email. Linda had heard of similar programs that offered many benefits to seniors aside from just learning how to use the computer, including increased connectivity to family and friends, increased empowerment and autonomy, and access to information about health and activities. She saw the Senior Cyber Café initiative as a vital component of the socialization programs offered by the agency in its partnership with senior centers.

Linda reviewed her notes on the complaints. She was sensitive to the seniors' concerns as she recognized that many of them were adapting to "aging," as she had learned in her gerontology training. Some of the class participants might even feel embarrassed over their sense of helplessness with computers and the Internet. In terms of the complaints, apparently during the classes Kim and Mark came across as condescending to the seniors. For instance, one senior complained that Kim had a patronizing attitude when she answered their questions and tended to dismiss their concerns, often replying "why?" Another senior said that Mark sometimes acted like they were mentally impaired, overcompensating when he spoke to them and showed them how to use the applications. These behaviors were interfering with the seniors' enjoyment and their patience in the learning process. Enthusiasm for the classes was high—there was already a waiting list for the next class session when the current one ended in eight weeks—and Linda didn't want anything to jeopardize it.

Background

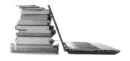

The Mid Florida Area Agency on Aging office in Gainesville is one of 11 Area Agencies on Aging (AAA) in Florida. The AAAs are private nonprofit entities that plan, coordinate, and fund support services for seniors in their respective services areas. They are an integral component of the elder services network of the Florida Department of Elder Affairs, the designated State Unit on Aging, which was created by the Older Americans Act of 1965. Through partnerships with local agencies, faith-based and nonprofit community organizations, and local governments, the AAAs deliver an array of services to residents age 60 and older to continue to live active, healthy lives in their senior years.

One of the most important partnerships for the AAAs is with Florida's senior centers. The senior centers are community facilities that provide a broad range of educational, recreational, and wellness services to independent seniors. They provide seniors with the opportunity to join together to visit with friends and participate in community-based activities. The majority of senior centers are located in free-standing buildings, within community or recreation centers, or in local government buildings. The senior centers use their own funds to operate and as a result must rely heavily on volunteers. Florida, with one of the largest concentrations of residents age 60 and older, has approximately 260 senior centers, which draw approximately 380,000 visitors per year and more than 18,500 visitors per day.[1]

Next Steps

Linda evaluated her alternatives. She recognized that with budget constraints public organizations like her agency and the senior centers needed the time and skills of volunteers. The success of the Senior Cyber Café program was important to her agency and she needed to ensure she had volunteers with the necessary computer skills to teach the classes. However, she also recognized that many of these volunteers, including Kim and Mark, did not have any formal training or experience in teaching, especially to senior citizens.

Given the existing complaints, Linda realized that she may need to replace Kim and Mark as instructors. This action might set a good example to other volunteers that they need to be more sensitive in how they interact with seniors. However, this action will be difficult to implement as she doesn't have many other volunteers with their level of computer proficiency and she doesn't want to interrupt the class sessions. Moreover, it might backfire on the agency by giving a negative impression for other volunteers, especially if Kim and Mark react poorly to the decision. Kim and Mark may be well-intentioned and may simply not be aware of their offensive communication behaviors. Linda recognized that intergenerational communication was often based on stereotypical expectations. She didn't want to overreact, and replacing them might send the wrong signal. Linda wanted to create an enjoyable experience for volunteers so they would continue to come back as well as encourage others to volunteer through positive word-of-mouth.

Another alternative might be to move Kim and Mark into another role that did not require teaching or direct interaction with the seniors in the class. Again, this might be difficult as she did not have many other volunteers with the same computer skills. She could not afford to hire professional computer trainers to teach the Senior Cyber Café project given budget constraints. In addition, it would be hard to find an alternate role in the agency that did not involve direct interaction with seniors at least on some level. Another option might be to pair a staff member or a more senior volunteer with Kim and Mark in the classroom to offer some mentoring. Linda even considered a more far-reaching solution—offer an age-sensitive communication training program for all volunteers. Linda weighed her alternatives. She needed to make a decision before next week's class at the senior center.

Discussion Questions

1. How would you respond to the complaints?

2. Would you replace Kim and Mark as instructors for the classes?

3. Explain what intergenerational communication issues may be present? How would you manage them?

4. Describe the challenges of managing and motivating volunteers within the public health workforce.

Reference

[1] Florida Department of Elder Affairs. (2010, November 20). *Florida's Senior Centers*. Retrieved from http://elderaffairs.state.fl.us/english/seniorcenter.php

Case 64

CASE CONTRIBUTOR **Scott D. Musch**

Situation

Ryan, the chief of the state's Bureau of Lead Poisoning Prevention, has received numerous calls, emails, and letters from concerned parents of young children after the recent recall of toys found to contain lead-based paint. The toys were imported by a well-known U.S. company from its contract manufacturer in China. The company, in coordination with the U.S. Consumer Product Safety Commission, announced the recall last month. The toys represented a very small fraction of the company's overall business and product line, so there seemed to be a perception of the lack of urgency in dealing with the recall. Parents have been outraged, not just about the possibility of lead poisoning, but frustrated over how the company is dealing with the problem. The company has refused all interview requests and has issued one brief statement saying an investigation is underway and "We are implementing a corrective action plan." No other details have been offered. Parents are angry as they feel the company is keeping them in the dark as the recall applied to only one of its many toy product lines that are popular with young children. Parents want to know what the corrective action plan reveals. In addition, how safe are the company's other products? Is a recall coming?

Ryan is concerned by the company's insufficient communication strategy both with his agency and the general public. His calls to the company's executive office have been returned with simple, prepared statements that offer no additional insight. He did manage to connect with an employee within the company through an old networking contact. The employee revealed that he hasn't seen any internal communications via email or memo on the issue. The employee really didn't know what was going on with the company's management team and why they have been so silent. Ryan joined the parent's frustration. His primary concern is to protect the well-being and safety of the state's children. Without the company's cooperation, however, he cannot perform his job.

Background

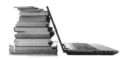

Lead exposure in American children has fallen significantly in the last several decades after concerted efforts by public health officials to reduce exposure among children from lead-based paint and lead-contaminated dust in deteriorating buildings. Despite this progress, renewed concern has emerged from exposure to products containing lead that have been imported from developing countries, namely China. Lead poisoning in children causes learning disabilities, kidney failure, anemia, and irreversible brain damage. The U.S. Consumer Product Safety Commission (CPSC) has announced the recall of numerous children's products containing hazardous amounts of lead imported from China over the last several years, including metal jewelry, toys, gloves, and chalk.

The CPSC is an independent federal regulatory agency created in 1972 by Congress under the Consumer Product Safety Act. The CPSC protects the public from unreasonable risks of injury or death from consumer products that pose a fire, electrical, chemical, or mechanical hazard or that can injure children. The Federal Hazardous Substances Act (FHSA) requires that certain hazardous household products are labeled to alert consumers to potential hazards and to inform them of measures they need to protect themselves from those hazards. The FHSA gives the CPSC the authority to ban any hazardous substance if it determines that the product is so hazardous that the labeling required by the act is inadequate to protect the public. Under the FHSA, any toy or other article that is intended for use by children and that contains a hazardous substance is banned if a child can gain access to the substance.

The American public is growing increasingly concerned over the safety of products imported from China. Recent headline stories of Chinese scandals, involving pet food poisonings, bacterial parasites in contact lens solutions, and deadly toothpaste containing a solvent used in antifreeze, have only contributed to the alarm. Although inspected and banned if necessary, not all products containing hazardous materials are discovered before making it into the American marketplace. The ultimate responsibility for this exposure to hazardous contaminants lies with U.S. companies purchasing the foreign products.

Next Steps

Ryan weighs his options on how to respond to the company's insufficient communication and at the same time protect the public from any additional exposure to lead poisoning. He needs to coordinate an effective approach by drawing on federal and state agencies, the media, consumer advocates, and even the group of outraged parents.

Discussion Questions

1. What are the most pressing problems for Ryan?

2. What steps could Ryan take to encourage the company to communicate more openly with his agency and the public?

3. Aside from the announced recall, does the company have any further obligation or ethical responsibility to provide additional information to the public?

4. The employee within the company revealed that he had not seen any internal communication about the recall and public response. What does this suggest about the company's organizational communication?

5. If you were an executive at the company, how would you deal with this situation?

6. As the executive, how would your response vary according to the audience—federal and state agencies, the media, consumer advocates, and parents?

Case 65 | A Communications Challenge

CASE CONTRIBUTOR **Kathleen M. Reville**

Situation

Susan Spencer, the human resources director for the Center for Human Services (CHS), was reviewing the most recent employee satisfaction survey results and was worried. The results, gathered every two years, continued to show a frustration with communication among CHS's largest workforce, those who provide direct service to individuals with disabilities. These staff felt that they weren't getting the information they needed and felt disconnected from the organization. These results were troubling because the organization had recently invested a substantial amount of money in its communication efforts including doubling the size of staff, upgrading technology, and increasing printed collateral. Why wasn't this information reaching these staff members?

Background

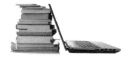

CHS is a nonprofit, full-service health and human services agency that has experienced profound growth over the last 10 years, growing from an $8 million budget to a $150+ million budget. This rapid growth was the result of the acquisitions of other non-profit agencies, each of which continued to function independently. This culture of independence created silos, with each affiliate organization struggling to understand its role within the larger whole. A new internal communication strategy must be developed for CHS that will enable it to communicate effectively throughout all levels of the organization.

CHS employs 3400 staff members who represent a variety of clinical and professional arenas. The services provided by CHS include residential care for adults with developmental disabilities, pediatric long-term and subacute care, mental health and substance abuse services, day habilitation and adult day health programs, residential programs, and schools for behaviorally challenged children.

The majority of staff is represented by individuals who speak English as a second language and who have not advanced beyond a high school degree. Many of these staff do not own computers and do not have access to email. These staff, known as direct service professionals (DSPs), are also a target for union activity, which has increased within the health and human services sector and for which CHS is a target. If this workforce is to be happily engaged at CHS, they must be aware of the important work of the organization and their role in the accomplishment of this work.

Next Steps

Susan must work quickly with the Communications Office to develop a strategy to reach the DSP workforce. She has an ample budget, but must find ways to reach audiences of varying levels of sophistication and reading ability.

Discussion Questions

1. What methods of communication would you suggest be part of the overall strategy?

2. How should managers be drawn into this internal plan? What is the role of management and how should this role be monitored?

3. How will Susan determine whether her new strategies are effective?

Case 66

Ethical Limits of Patient Satisfaction

CASE CONTRIBUTOR Krystina Cunningham

Situation

A patient was admitted to an inpatient rehabilitation center following a lengthy hospital stay after sustaining a cervical level spinal cord injury and compound tibial fracture in a motor vehicle accident. The inpatient rehabilitation center is a transitional hospital that focuses on therapy services (physical therapy, occupational therapy, respiratory therapy, and speech-language pathology). The patient's spinal cord injury resulted in tetraplegia, impairment in motor function in all four limbs, requiring significant assistance with all activities of daily living. In addition, the compound tibial fracture required the patient to have a bulky external fixator, which is a device comprising a metal splint and metal supports that are drilled into the patient's bone for stability until healing is complete.

Due to the status of the patient's family in the community, the patient was admitted with a "high profile" VIP (very important person) status. The therapists and staff were advised that the patient's family selected the rehabilitation center based on recent publicity promoting therapy services capable of enhancing recovery following spinal cord injury. The patient's sister was planning a wedding, and the patient and his family were hoping that the patient would be capable of walking down the aisle during the ceremony.

During the first two months of his admission, therapists worked with the patient to improve his sitting balance and self-care. The patient trialed a power wheelchair, but due to fatigue, the patient was unsafe to drive the wheelchair without constant supervision. The patient made very little progress due to complaints of pain, fatigue, and an upset stomach; refusal to begin therapy before noon; late arrival to all therapy sessions due to skewed personal priorities; and eventually, the development of pneumonia and the medical complications associated with pneumonia. With the development of pneumonia, the patient was returned to acute care for medical management.

When the patient was medically stable for transfer back to inpatient rehabilitation, the admitting physician denied the patient due to the limited progress made during the patient's initial stay. However, due to the patient's VIP status and positive health insurance coverage, the hospital administrators encouraged the physician to resume services. The physician submitted to the request and admitted the patient back to inpatient rehabilitation.

Problems continued to occur with the patient's participation and progress in therapy. However, the patient began asking his therapists to train his family and friends to assist with transfer to/from a car so he could leave the hospital to attend his sister's wedding. The physician denied this request stating that riding in the car was not safe at this time due to the patient's current condition and co-morbidities. The physician did recommend that the insurance company hire a transport service to pick the patient up in a full-sized van equipped to transport the patient within his wheelchair.

After agreeing to the wheelchair transport van, the patient demanded that he be in control of his own mobility at the wedding and reception, and thus was requesting the use of a power wheelchair. The occupational therapist agreed to trial a power wheelchair with the patient and to train him how to manage all controls and set-up of the wheelchair if, and only if, he agreed to be ready for therapy at the scheduled time and participate during a full session. However, by the time the patient began participating regularly in therapy sessions, the therapists had less than one week to prepare for the event.

The patient and his family were requesting that he be ready to leave the hospital at 8 a.m. for prewedding events. The patient wanted to stay for the duration of the reception and return to the hospital by midnight. Hospital regulations allow leave from the hospital for a maximum of 8 hours (leaving at 9 a.m. after medication administration and returning by 6 p.m. in time for evening medication administration and dinner). Following complaints made by the patient and his family to the hospital's administrators, the duration for his leave was granted. For this reason, the nursing staff and therapists had to prepare the family to administer medications; administer IV antibiotics; assist with changing the patient's brief (adult diaper) in the case of a bowel or bladder accident; assist the patient with intermittent catheterization (required every 3–4 hours to empty the patient's bladder); assist with pressure relief by tilting the patient back in his chair for 15 minutes every hour to prevent pressure ulcers; and transfer the patient to/from a bed to allow for changing his brief in the case of an accident.

The patient's family was not able to manage all of these needs, so the patient's insurance company hired a nurse and her assistant to perform all nursing duties and assist with transfers. The nurses planned to rent a hospital bed to be transported to the reception hall and set up in a private room for availability to change the patient's brief and clothing as needed. Unfortunately, the only space the reception hall had available was a small coat closet that was not large enough for a hospital bed. Measurements were not taken of the reception hall, so it was also likely that the patient's wheelchair would not fit in the space.

Despite the therapists' report to the physician of the safety concerns regarding the proposed plan, the physician continued to entertain approval of the leave from the hospital. The nursing company provided a portable massage table that could be set up in the closet if needed. The physician requested that the therapists assess the safety after completing transfer training to this table. The nurse, her assistant, and the patient's father were then scheduled to attend therapy sessions to complete training to perform all tasks safely.

After training, the following concerns were reported to the patient and his caregivers and then the physician:

1. No measurements were taken for the space provided for set-up of the massage table. The therapists had no way to ensure that the massage table would fit into the space to be utilized if needed.

2. The patient had been unable to go more than 10 hours without a bowel accident over the past two weeks.

3. The massage table was only 3 feet wide and there were no bedrails/guardrails on the table to provide safety with rolling the patient (necessary in order to change his brief).

4. The external fixator stabilizing the patient's tibial fracture was compromised when the patient's caregivers were positioning him for transfers.

5. During transfers, the caregivers required more time than the therapists to perform the transfer due to their lack of practice, and the patient would get frustrated. As a result, the patient would begin yelling and rush the caregivers, putting the patient and the caregivers at risk for injury.

Next Steps

Due to these concerns, the physician reported to the patient and his family that his request for leave was being denied for the timeframe requested, but she offered to allow an eight-hour leave to avoid all of the above listed problems. The patient became irate, began yelling at the physician and therapists, and demanded to speak with the hospital administrators. To avoid such contact, the physician called a meeting alone with the therapists in an attempt to find a compromise to the patient's demands.

Discussion Questions

1. The physician has the final decision with regard to granting or denying a leave of absence and the terms of that leave. With pressure from administration and the patient and strong recommendations against the leave from the therapists, what would you do if you were the physician?

2. It is very important to the patient and his family to be part of his sister's wedding. The family even postponed the wedding after the patient's initial accident to allow him time to stabilize medically in order for him to leave the hospital to attend. How would you, as a therapist, have handled the situation?

3. How would you as a health administrator mitigate the situation to please your customer (the patient and his family), the physician, and your employees (the therapists and nurses)?

4. Should the rules/policies of a hospital be flexible to appease a patient and/or patient's family? If so, in what situations and at whose discretion? If the policies were upheld, how would that have changed the situation?

5. Accidents occur when a chain of errors occur, a series of poor decisions are made, or policies put in place for safety are ignored. What are potential negative outcomes if the patient were allowed to leave the hospital under these circumstances? Are these consequences worth the risk?

Case 67

CASE CONTRIBUTOR **Kevin Wiley, Jr.**

Situation

Action on Disease, Development, and Sustainability (ADDS), a nongovernmental organization (NGO) operating in Southeast Asia, is committed to improving water systems in marginalized communities across Thailand, Cambodia, and Laos. ADDS is predominantly funded by the World Health Organization (WHO) and the University of South-East Asia. ADDS has been a major contributor in reducing the incidence of waterborne disease near the northeastern border of Thailand, specifically schistosomiasis. Schistosomiasis, caused by parasitic worms, is considered a neglected tropical disease (NTD) transmitted while bathing, swimming, or wading in contaminated water. The disease can persist in the brain or spinal cord, causing seizures, paralysis, or spinal cord inflammation.

The WHO conducts biannual evaluations of ADDS programs, requiring that the NGO submit detailed incidence and financial reports. Dr. Daniel Inglehart, the director of ADDS Department of Neglected Disease, is instructed by the Thailand Ministry of Health (MOH) to withhold disease incidence reports because an exorbitant tourist season is expected. The WHO publishes information about the health status of Thailand provided by ADDS; furthermore, these reports are required for the continuation of funding from the WHO. The deadline to submit is in five days and Dr. Inglehart must receive approval from the MOH to release this information. Dr. Inglehart has yet to receive approval. Essential resources for ADDS's many ongoing programs are at stake if there is a failure to comply with WHO's guidelines. The MOH has also informed Dr. Inglehart that if the report is published, ADDS will no longer be able to conduct operations in Thailand.

Background

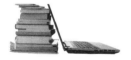

Most NTD-related infections can be reduced or eliminated by controlling vectors that transmit these diseases through improved sanitation, living conditions, and water systems. Many common NTDs are found in Asia, Africa, and Latin America, including Dengue fever, leishmaniasis, leprosy, Guinea worm disease, and rabies. These diseases disproportionately affect impoverished populations around the world in areas where access to clean water and proper human waste disposal remain nonexistent.

Next Steps

The request and threats by the MOH have put Dr. Inglehart in a financial and ethical dilemma. Dr. Inglehart has prepared the report but has yet to send it to the WHO. He appealed to the MOH with no avail. Dr. Inglehart has two days before the WHO deadline lapses.

Discussion Questions

1. What concessions could Dr. Inglehart and WHO representatives make in future negotiations with the MOH to ensure timely report submission/publication without any disruption to the highly profitable tourist season?

2. How should Dr. Inglehart respond if the MOH requests that he withhold reports in the future?

3. If the WHO were to stop funding this program in Southeast Asia, what are some possible repercussions for WHO in the region? For ADDS?

4. Dr. Inglehart could seek funding from other institutions across the globe, but none as prestigious or reputable as the WHO. How could severing ties with the WHO affect ADDS's relationship with the international public health community?

Case 68

A Friend's Dilemma

CASE CONTRIBUTOR Scott D. Musch

Situation

Stacy is an administrative assistant at the Los Angeles-Downtown Wellness Center, an HIV testing site funded by the California Department of Public Health (CDPH). In addition to HIV testing, the Wellness Center provides HIV prevention education services, HIV/AIDS medical treatment, and HIV support services such as case management and counseling. Stacy's job primarily involves data entry and processing. Her main responsibility is to assist in filling out the HIV/AIDS case report forms required by the CDPH for confirmed HIV tests.

Although she has worked at the Wellness Center for only eight months, she enjoys the work and recognizes the highly sensitive nature of her job. In the course of her work, she handles patient medical record files and sees the names of patients who have tested positive for HIV. Given the routine of her work, she typically processes the information without much thought to patient names, until this afternoon. In the patient file she is holding, she recognizes the name—Eric—her best friend's boyfriend. He tested positive for HIV and gonorrhea. Linda, her best friend, has been dating Eric exclusively for the last year and she believes that Linda has not had sexual relations with anyone else during that time.

Background

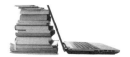

The Wellness Center is administered by a county health department and operates pursuant to the California Health and Safety Code. The Health and Safety Code (Section 121022[a]) requires healthcare providers and clinical laboratories to report HIV infection by patient name to the local health officer and mandates local health officers to report HIV cases by patient name to the CDPH. The report consists of a completed copy of a HIV/AIDS case report form, which is coordinated with the CDPH, Office of AIDS, HIV/AIDS Case Registry. Prior to 2007, patient names were not reported. In 2007, the California Department of Health repealed non-name code and partial non-name code used for HIV reporting and required healthcare providers, laboratories, and local health officers to use patient names when reporting cases of HIV infection.[1] This change decreased the reporting burden for reporting entities and the name-based HIV reporting system ensured that California remained eligible for federal funding.

All local health department employees and contractors with access to confidential HIV-related information are required to sign a confidentiality agreement form that informs staff of the penalties associated with a breach of confidentiality as well as the procedures for reporting a breach. As an employee of the Wellness Center, Stacy signed a confidentiality agreement form prior to being allowed to handle confidential HIV-related health records. In addition, Stacy attended a mandatory Data and Security Training session offered to new staff who will handle patient data entry. The training program outlined the policies and procedures of maintaining confidentiality. During the training, Stacy learned that any person who willfully, maliciously, or negligently discloses the content of any confidential public health record to a third party, except in accordance to a written authorization or as authorized by law, can be subject to civil and criminal penalties, including imprisonment.

Next Steps

After entering Eric's information into the case report form, Stacy reaches for the telephone to call Linda but then stops to think. Stacy knows that Eric isn't the type of person who will tell Linda and admit his infidelity. If Stacy tells Linda, she will be upset and will confront Eric. Eric will try to figure out how Linda found out about his test and will likely inquire at the Wellness Center, which might lead back to Stacy. If the Wellness Center's administrator finds out, Stacy will be terminated and could face additional penalties. But is her job worth the risk of potentially putting her friend's health in jeopardy?

Discussion Questions

1. What should Stacy do in her situation?

2. Does the confidentiality protection facilitate or inhibit the interests of public health when involving infectious diseases?

3. How will Stacy's supervisor handle a breach of confidentiality?

4. If you were Stacy's supervisor and she asked for your advice, what would you recommend?

Reference

[1] California Department of Public Health. (n.d.). R-06-014E-Reporting HIV infection by name. Retrieved from http://www.cdph.ca.gov/services/DPOPP/regs/Pages/R-06-014E-ReportingHIVInfectionbyName.aspx

Case 69 | Stolen Briefcase

CASE CONTRIBUTOR **Scott D. Musch**

Situation

After two years as a disease intervention specialist for the Texas Department of State Health Services—Infectious Disease Control Unit, Carlos was aware of the many challenges associated with his job. Although the title doesn't sound dangerous, the job can be at times. His responsibilities include not only informing people who test positive for sexually transmitted diseases (STDs), including HIV, but also tracking down their sex partners. These situations can become confrontational, particularly when working with marginal information and dealing with irate people who don't want to face the news. Today, however, didn't involve any confrontations, but rather something more serious. After finishing a field visit in an economically depressed inner-city neighborhood, Carlos returned to his car to find the passenger door window broken, door ajar, and his briefcase containing case interview files missing.

Background

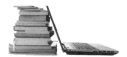

A disease intervention specialist (DIS) is a trained public health professional who is responsible for finding and counseling patients, sex partners, and others suspected of having an STD or other communicable disease. The main objective of this frontline public health work is to prevent and control disease transmission by ensuring that all people who have been diagnosed or exposed to a communicable disease are promptly examined and adequately treated. Among his or her many duties, the DIS conducts field visits to locate, motivate, and refer communicable disease patients and their partners/contacts for medical evaluation and treatment at public or private healthcare providers. Given the sensitive and personal nature of STD information, the DIS must follow a strict protocol to maintain confidentiality.

The DIS has the responsibility to ensure that persons who are infected with an STD, or who are at risk of acquiring an STD, receive appropriate medical care at the earliest possible time. Although reaching a person by the telephone for initial follow-up activities is permitted, it is not the preferred method for in-depth investigation and dealing with highly sensitive issues such as HIV or HIV-partner notification. A field call is the most effective follow-up method and frequently the most efficient. The Texas Department of State Health Services has an established set of operating procedures and standards (HIV/STD Public Health Follow-Up Confidential Information Security Procedures) for all HIV/STD field and support staff involving the handling of confidential information.[1] The department's local responsible party (LRP) implements and enforces these policies and procedures, which are designed in part to ensure that the DIS observes certain safeguards to protect the nature of his or her professional capacity and the privacy of individuals in the course of disease intervention activities. The LRP also has the responsibility of reporting and assisting in investigating breaches. Some of the standard procedures for field visits include:

- Field visits need to be conducted in unmarked vehicles to ensure client confidentiality.
- Field records containing confidential information are not to be left unattended outside the office.
- Documents used in the field should contain the minimum amount of confidential information necessary to conduct the field investigation.
- Contents of field records should not be divulged to any unauthorized persons.
- Field records should be properly coded, and code sheets should not be kept in the same container as the field records.

Next Steps

Carlos planned multiple calls today to make the most efficient use of his field time. His briefcase contained a number of files that contained information to identify the addresses and names of people in the neighborhood whom he planned to visit. Although the field records were coded, there were other papers in his briefcase that would make it obvious in what capacity he was working. Carlos had locked the files in his briefcase after reviewing them, placed the briefcase under the passenger seat, and locked the car before heading off to his first client's apartment. Although he knew this neighborhood had a high crime rate, he thought his car would be safe parked on the street. After all, his briefcase wasn't even visible.

Discussion Questions

1. How should Carlos handle this situation?

2. Did Carlos violate any operating procedures?

3. What should the LRP do in this situation?

Reference

[1] Texas Department of State Health Services. (2010, September 28). HIV/STD security policies and procedures. Retrieved from http://www.dshs.state.tx.us/hivstd/policy/security.shtm

Case 70

Theatre of Operation—Transplant Solutions in Public Health

CASE CONTRIBUTOR **Adam Miller**

Situation

As the snow fell gently outside his office window, Nathan couldn't help but take a minute to enjoy the wintery scene. The snow had been coming since early morning when he arrived, and by now had turned the cold and grey city below into a bright and renewed winter wonderland. It seemed so peaceful, he thought. It was in such contrast to the current swirl of thoughts on his mind regarding the unusual events unfolding in his office. It was only 10:30 a.m., and due to the numerous calls, questions, and decisions to be made, even his coffee cup seemed to be heavier than usual today. He rapped his fingers on the side of the warm mug, still engrossed in the peaceful scene beyond his window, diverting his attention.

"The Secretary is on the line for you, Nathan," said Laura, his department's administrative assistant, as she opened his office door. "Would you like me to put her through?" she asked. And with that, the momentary seasonal sabbatical was abruptly ended, and Nathan returned to the present and the situation at hand.

Nathan Austin was the most recent leadership addition to the state Department of Health, recently appointed Director of Policy—Health Care Statistics and Standards. Even though the job was outside of his traditional area of expertise (he was a trained epidemiologist), budget cuts and personnel reductions in both departments had necessitated his appointment. With the most recent recession, the state government had cut almost 5% of its workforce, many of whom were employees in specialized functional areas.

With an MPH degree from a highly respected university and a varied background in public health subjects, Nathan had felt more excited than apprehensive to take the new position, even though he knew it would require significantly more skill in dealing with people and ambiguity than his previous role. Many people viewed his position as their "gateway" to certain areas of expertise within the department, kind of a "jack of all trades" regarding policy in specialized areas that had diffuse or less-than-evident contact points. Additionally, in the few months he had been in the department, he had already realized that he would often have to "make the tough call" in his new role—being the final say on important and rapid developing matters, often without complete information and in subject areas that were not his most comfortable areas of expertise.

The situation unfolding currently was a perfect example of this new responsibility. When he arrived at his office this morning, a local mayor had called the Secretary of Health for assistance regarding a young girl in his municipality who had been matched with a living donor for a kidney transplant. Arrangements were currently underway at the local university hospital for the procedure, which had an excellent reputation for the needed procedure. Unfortunately, a number of issues had surfaced that were making what seemed like a simple, heartwarming story a far more complex issue. The Secretary has requested that Nathan intervene and assist the parties in finding a "workable and practical solution."

After initial review of the situation, Nathan had found out that the young girl was in the United States possibly as a refugee, though her status may have recently expired. Further, the current legal resident and/or refugee status of her parents could not be verified, and linguistic barriers were presenting issues for everyone involved. While the medical team on the ground was certain that they could perform the surgery, the hospital administration wanted to make sure both federal and state laws were followed. All parties had requested that verification be made, though they were having difficulty isolating exactly what they needed and from whom, which was creating a critical time delay in both administrative and medical preparations.

Further complicating matters was the process of ensuring that the many medications needed posttransplant were available for the young girl following her surgery. Under most circumstances, patients must demonstrate an ability to pay for their medication, either through a third party or themselves, in order to receive an organ transplant. And while all of the pharmaceutical companies had been very willing to help the girl in need, a variety of issues had to be resolved; some companies had policies that would allow them to give only to individuals in the country legally and others were concerned that her future residency status may present an issue. Their U.S.-based patient assistance programs could not easily extend beyond U.S. borders and they could not guarantee medication assistance in all circumstances if she returned to her home country. It was determined that these issues would have to be resolved in order for the transplant to proceed, and the parties were not in agreement on how to achieve this end.

To make matters even more complicated, time was becoming an issue for making a decision on the transplant—and Nathan was finding direct and timely answers to the questions at hand more difficult by the moment. While not directly in charge of the decision-making processes, his assistance had been requested and his ability to manage the situation and find solutions for all parties involved would play a critical—even decisive—role in the outcome. Perhaps if he had a few days, or even a week, he would be confident he had all the data and confirmations he needed to make a final decision and provide recommendations. He didn't have the power to mandate action and didn't want to spend undue amounts of time to re-create the wheel on this, but so far the parties had yet to come to a consensus on practical or policy matters.

But, it appeared that he would have to make a call on how to proceed, and from the large stack of calls, texts, and emails from an ever-growing, concerned list of parties, which by now included prominent state elected officials, and even the local media, his decisions and their outcomes would be monitored closely.

Background

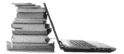

The desire to successfully achieve organ transplantation in medicine is an ancient one, with Chinese texts speaking to the concept of organ transplantation in the fourth century B.C.[1] Since that time, there have been a number of advances in the science of organ transplantation. Since the first living-related kidney transplant between identical twins in 1954 by Drs. Joseph Murray and John Harrison at Peter Bent Brigham Hospital in Boston Massachusetts, advances in the science of organ transplantation have come at a steady pace.[2] From early experiments, advances in tissue typing, anti-rejection treatments, and organ preservation, among many others, have allowed the field of organ transplantation to mature significantly.[3]

Due to medical advances in the treatment of many chronic diseases, the need for organ transplantation has steadily outpaced the available supply of organs. As of January 2011, approximately 101,000 people in the United States were waiting for an organ transplant.[4] And while the organ transplant list grows by 300 each month, each day 19 people die waiting for an organ transplant due to the limited supply of organs.[5] This disparity between supply and demand for such organs has produced much moral and ethical debate on the issue, creating the need for both law and policy development. Further, the complex and overlapping legal and regulatory environment unrelated to the development of organ transplantation (or medicine in general) may present unforeseen or difficult-to-solve complexities within certain situations.

As organ donation is a deeply personal gift, federal law has been passed to manage this process. Laws such as the 1984 National Organ Transplant Act established the Organ Procurement and Transplant Network (OPTN), a national organ sharing system to guarantee, among other things, fairness in the allocation of organs for transplant.[6] Other prominent laws include the 1987 Uniform Anatomical Gift Act and the 1991 Patient Self-Determination Act.[7] State governments have also played an active role in the management of organ transplantation, most actively in the areas of state anatomical gift acts, informed and other consent acts, organ donation education, as well as issues pertaining to advance directives.

The field of public health has certainly not been silent on the issue of organ transplantation and related issues. Public health officials are deeply involved in all aspects of the issue, including the policy and regulatory environment, and are actively helping to provide many means of expertise and assistance. Innovations concerning organ transplantation involving the field of public health are evident around the country and within all levels of government. One example includes the Massachusetts Organ Donation Initiative, a statewide effort to reduce the disparity between available organ supply and demand that included a unique partnership among organ procurement organizations, major teaching hospitals, and the state's department of public health.[8]

Those involved in the field of public health will continue to play a pivotal role in the future of policy formation regarding organ transplantation and associated issues, and will need to engage and advise many parties. Complexities abound, however, and may manifest in a variety of manners, including politically, fiscally, or operationally. For example, the

Arizona Health Care Cost Containment System has potentially stopped funding for certain types of transplants, citing an established low probability of success and a deteriorating state fiscal environment.[9] Each public health official involved with issues such as transplantation will face a growing number of internal and external challenges that must be managed successfully in order to achieve important goals.

Next Steps

As Nathan quickly put down his coffee mug, he knew he would like a few more minutes to re-analyze his thoughts and call the Secretary back, but she would want an answer immediately as to his plans to proceed. As he reflected on the events of the morning in his mind, he had been given little time to plan, but the outcome of his actions would most likely affect a number of people. He would have to use his collective skills, as well as the minds around him, to find a successful path to his goal of helping those who had reached out this morning.

With his action plan outline in hand that he had carefully written in preparation for this call, Nathan looked up from his desk and gave a nod to Laura. "Please put the Secretary through."

Discussion Questions

1. How would you proceed if you were Nathan? What would you say to the Secretary?

2. What are the issues to be resolved? In what order? What are the most reasonable potential solutions?

3. What is the responsibility of a public health official in the political process? What types of skills are needed in these situations? How do you successfully deploy them?

4. Does an individual in this situation have a responsibility to ensure that all information has been considered before making a decision? Why or why not?

5. Should public health officials take a position concerning organ transplantation for individuals without documentation? What types of moral hazards are potentially involved?

References

[1] The Gift of a Lifetime. (2004). *History of transplantation—Timeline*. Retrieved from http://www.organtransplants.org/understanding/history/

[2] United Network for Organ Sharing. (2011). *History of organ donation*. Retrieved from http://www.unos.org/donation/index.php?topic=history

[3] Fix, M. (n.d.). *Kidney transplantation: Past, present and future—History*. Stanford University. [Class Project]. Retrieved from http://www.stanford.edu/dept/HPS/transplant/html/history.html

4. U.S. Department of Health and Human Services, Organ Procurement and Transplantation Network. (2011). *In Data*. Retrieved from http://optn.transplant.hrsa.gov/

5. The Mayo Clinic. (n.d.). Organ Donation. In *Transplant Programs at Mayo Clinic*. Retrieved from http://www.mayoclinic.org/transplant/organ-donation.html

6. Cengage, G. (2003). Organ Donation. In *Encyclopedia of Everyday Law. eNotes.com*. (Ed. Shirelle Phelps). Retrieved from http://www.enotes.com/everyday-law-encyclopedia/organ-donation

7. The Gift of a Lifetime. (2004). *Understanding donation*. Retrieved from http://www.organtransplants.org/understanding/unos/

8. Koh, H. K., Jacobson, M. D., Lyddy, A. M., O'Connor, K. J., Fitzpatrick, S. M., Krakow, M., . . . Luskin, R. S. (2007). A statewide public health approach to improving organ donation: the Massachusetts Organ Donation Initiative. *American Journal of Public Health*, *97*(1), 30–36. doi: 10.2105/AJPH.2005.077701

9. Tripp, K. (2011, February 3). *Republicans stand firm on AHCCCS transplant funding*. Retrieved from http://ktar.com/category/local-news-articles/20110203/Republicans-stand-firm-on-AHCCCS-transplant-funding/

Case 71

Role of Public Health in End-of-Life Issues

CASE CONTRIBUTOR **William G. Wuenstel**

Situation

Fred is an 87-year-old who resides with his wife in a senior retirement community in Florida after spending most of his adult life in Ohio. Even though his adult children still live in the North, they retain their close family ties with frequent phone calls and vacation visits. Fred maintains an active lifestyle by participating in the community activities including the fitness center and walking trails, and his health status has been labeled "good" by his wife. He is under the care of a family physician whom he sees regularly for routine checkups including his blood pressure and labs drawn for cholesterol and other screening levels. The only prescribed medications that Fred takes are for the treatment of his hypertension and hypercholesterolemia and according to his wife, they both take numerous vitamin and herbal supplements. In addition, Fred receives his annual flu vaccination.

Since Fred was considered in good health and often was told that by the healthcare providers that he was a young 87-year-old, it came as a surprise to his wife and family when Fred suffered a cardiac event. It happened during the early morning hours after having a restless night. Fred experienced an upset stomach along with nausea and general upper body pain. He took an over-the-counter antacid and attempted to return to sleep. He reported that the pain continued but appeared to be lessening during the night. In the morning upon wakening he sat on the edge of the bed and called his wife, for the pain had suddenly become intolerable. As his wife assisted him from the edge of the bed, Fred suddenly grabbed his chest and yelled out, collapsing onto the bedroom floor. Fred's wife quickly called 911.

The Fire and Rescue station is located close to the senior community where Fred lives and responded within minutes. When the paramedics arrived, Fred's wife was in the process of performing CPR. The paramedics immediately assessed Fred and determined to intervene with supplement oxygen, and the defibrillation of Fred's heart. After several attempts, Fred's heart rhythm returned but was irregular. Intravenous fluids were administered to assist with his blood pressure and Fred was transported to the closest hospital.

Fred spent very little time in the emergency department of the hospital as arrangements were already made for him to be admitted to the cardiac intensive care unit. The team of nurses and the intensivist were on standby and quickly assessed his condition, preparing him for a cardiac intervention that would include a study of his cardiac vessels, possible reopening of a cardiac vessel, and the possible insertion of a stent. During the procedure, Fred suffered another cardiac event but was successfully resuscitated. He returned to the cardiac intensive care unit under sedation, and was carefully monitored throughout the night.

During the next two days, Fred's response to medication was considered problematic. His blood pressure was low requiring intravenous fluids and medications, his heart rhythm was irregular intermittently, and his urine output was rapidly decreasing. On the night of his third day, Fred suffered a stroke, which impaired his ability to breathe on his own. Ventilator supports along with additional intravenous medications were administered to keep Fred stable. Fred's family had arrived from out of town and with their mother they kept vigil at his bedside. The doctors on the case along with the nurses began to prepare the family for what was now considered a noncurative case. They pointed out to the family that Fred's kidneys had shut down and were no longer making urine. His heart had sustained too much damage to maintain adequate blood pressure, and now his lungs were beginning to fail, which all pointed to a domino of organ failure that would result in death. End-of-life care was introduced to the family by the social worker who conducts the public health role of transcending the continuum of care in various settings. Social workers accomplish this by providing a range of public health services that include health education, crisis intervention, supportive counseling, and case management.

Background

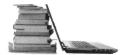

End-of-life care issues are an everyday occurrence in most intensive care units of hospitals. Yet, patients and families are unprepared to meet the medical emergency that can quickly change one's life even to the point of death. Agonizing decisions are made under the most difficult circumstances leading family members to be in conflict with other family members resulting in grief, anger, discord, and family breakup. With the increase in life expectancies, the aging population will achieve a greater proportion of chronic and debilitating terminal illnesses resulting in an increasing need to develop advance healthcare plans that include end-of-life care. According to the CDC, the impact of chronic diseases amounts to $325 billion in healthcare costs annually and contributes to four of every five deaths.[1]

According to the American Public Health Association (APHA), the goals of public health are in the promotion of health and disease prevention.[2] D'Onofrio and Ryndes from the School of Public Health at Berkeley contend that the promotion of health for the dying follows with the public health attempt to improve the quality of life.[3] In several APHA policy statements, the needless suffering and financial burden of nonbeneficial care was addressed with the patient's right to self-determination.[4] This right includes "the ability to express wishes in advance directive, to appoint a health care surrogate in making decisions when the patient is no longer able to do so, and to have these wishes honored by health care professionals."[5] There is a plethora of studies that have identified the frequency of deficiencies in providing care to the dying, including undertreatment of pain and ineffective communication between caregivers and patients and family members. The APHA's position on self-determination advocates the advance planning for end-of-life care through public education on the availability and the benefits of hospice as a method of promoting death with dignity.

Next Steps

Since Fred did not identify his advance directives or his medical preferences to his physician or to his family prior to his hospital stay, his wishes were unknown, resulting in uncertainty and confusion. Fred was orally intubated and connected to a ventilator that was providing life-sustaining oxygen and therefore unable to speak. In addition, the stroke had injured his brain and he was now considered brain dead. Multiple family meetings with nurses, the physician, chaplain, and social worker proceeded to explain the end-of-life medical options, but some of the family could not grasp and understand Fred's situation. These meetings became unbearable as individual members' opinions and beliefs on what they thought Fred would wish were in conflict with other members, leading to more confusion and stress. Fred's wife had to make the decisions since she was identified as the medical decision maker.

The main solution to resolving end-of-life issues is to develop advance healthcare plans up front as opposed to leaving emergency decisions to others. Plans would improve the quality of life for patients and their families who are facing the problems of physical care, psychosocial issues, and the spiritual needs by eliminating the struggles of being a burden to others, fears about death and dying, and unknown wishes.[6] This would begin with the prehospital care of identifying physicians and drug allergies, and knowing the location of important documents. Hospital care would involve identifying advance directives, family phone numbers, and determining the medical decision makers. Posthospital care would cover the needs for hospice care, organ-tissue donation plans, and burial plans.

Public health has been successful in protecting those most vulnerable from injury, disease, and negative health consequences.[3] Protection of children and youth has been a top priority due to the increased emphasis on pregnancy, perinatal health, and childhood illnesses while the special needs and vulnerability of people at the opposite end of age spectrum have been mostly ignored. A positive step in addressing this shortage would be to study the issues of bad dying and establish some type of statistical database.[3] Public health's role needs to include initiatives that support end-of-life care for people in the final stage of life; coordinate health care during this last phase by establishing cooperation among the various health-caregivers and organizations; develop education programs for professionals and public; support programs for family members; and lastly, establish metric measurements to improve outcomes.[7] Dying is the inevitable outcome of chronic diseases and illnesses and public health could contribute significantly to improving end-of-life care.

Discussion Questions

1. How can the social worker be helpful in this situation with Fred and his family?

2. What are the ethical issues that the healthcare providers and organization should consider as they manage this situation?

3. How can public health professionals engage society in discussing end-of-life issues?

4. What would be some of the most appropriate venues for such discussions and who should lead them?

5. In developing a surveillance model for addressing end-of-life issues, how can public health contribute?

6. Research suggests that public health can contribute to end-of-life care by studying the "epidemiology of bad dying." What questions about bad dying should be considered?

References

[1] Centers for Disease Control and Prevention (CDC). (2007, July 3). Assessment of chronic disease epidemiology workforce in State Health Departments – United States, 2003. *Preventing Chronic Disease, 4*(3). Retrieved from http://www.cdc.gov/ped/issues/2007/jul/06_0160.htm

[2] American Public Health Association (APHA). (n.d.). *What is public health?* Retrieved from http://www.apha.org/NR/rdonlyres/C5747B8-8682-4347-8DDF-A1E24E82B919/0/what_isPH_May1_Final.pdf

[3] D'Onofrio, C., & Ryndes, T. (n.d.). *The relevance of public health in improving access to end of life care.* Retrieved from http://www.growthouse.org/nhwg/essay5.htm

[4] American Public Health Association (APHA). (2005, December 14). *Supporting public health's role in addressing unmet needs at the end of life, policy number 2005-9.* Retrieved from http://www.apha.org/advocacy/policy/policysearch/default.htm?NRMODE=Published&N

[5] American Public Health Association (APHA). (2008, October 28). *Patients' rights to self-determination at the end of life, policy number 20086.* Retrieved from http://www.apha.org/advocacy/policy/policysearch/default.htm?NRMODE=Published&N

[6] Rao, J. K., Abraham, L. A., & Anderson, L. A. (2009, April). Novel approach, using end-of-life issues, for identifying items for public health surveillance. *Preventing Chronic Disease, 6*(2), 1–8. Retrieved from www.cdc.gov/pcd/issues/2009/apr/08_0120.htm

[7] Schneider, N., Lueckmann, S. L., Kuehne, F., Klindtworth, K., & Behman, M. (2010). Developing targets for public health initiatives to improve palliative care. *BMC Public Health, 10*(222), 1–9. Retrieved from http://www.biomedcentral.com/1471-2458/10/222

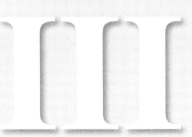

PART III

EXERCISES

Exercise 1 | Written Case Analysis

Following the sample outline provided in Figure 3–1, write an analysis of a case presented in the book. Alternatively, use the outline as a guide to formulate a new case scenario on a topical management issue in the healthcare industry.

Figure 3–1 Sample Outline for Written Case Analysis

I. Major Facts

Summarize the facts in narrative or outline form. These should include the most important and pertinent incidents in the situation. (Do not simply restate the entire case.)

II. Problem(s)

The facts of the case reveal one or more problems that require attention. Indicate those problems and briefly explain their importance.

III. Alternative Solutions and Probable Outcomes

A principle, "every action will have a reaction," pertains here. Analyze optional courses of action and the probable outcomes of each. This is one of the most important parts of the analysis. Remember that a decision not to act or to do nothing is always an alternative. However, doing nothing also has repercussions—sometimes worse repercussions than any other action. Identify as many alternatives as possible, even if some appear far-fetched.

IV. Recommended Solution and Probable Outcome

This section should include the recommended action, justification for the action, how that action would be implemented, and the probable outcome(s). While some of this information has been included in previous sections, it is still important to present the recommendation in its final form and to justify its selection.

Evaluation Criteria

Criteria for evaluation might include the following:
- Organization: Did the student answer all the parts of the assignment in a logical sequence?
- Integration: Did the student incorporate readings, including theories, research, and models, into the analysis?
- Management practice: Did the student consider several alternatives? What methods did the student present to assess the effectiveness of his/her decision(s)?
- Composition: Is the student's writing technically correct and stylistically appropriate?

Source: Kilpatrick, A. O., & Johnson, J. A. (1999). *Human Resources and Organizational Behavior: Cases in Health Services Management*. Chicago, IL: Health Administration Press.

Exercise 2 | Film Analysis and Discussion

View one or both of the films *Damaged Care* and/or *Contagion* while watching the human behavior dynamics, take note of the following:

1. Varying leadership styles
2. Ethical issues and decisions
3. Conflict management approaches
4. Examples of systems thinking
5. Power relationships and motivational dynamics

Bring your notes to class and share with others in small groups on each of the five topic areas.

Exercise 3 | SWOT Analysis

A SWOT analysis is a strategic planning exercise used to evaluate an organization's strengths, weaknesses, opportunities, and threats. The SWOT analysis should match the organization's resources and capabilities to the competitive environment in which it operates. The analysis should help guide the organization's formulation and selection of strategy. The SWOT analysis framework is often represented in a matrix, as shown in Figure 3–2.

Figure 3–2 SWOT Analysis Framework Matrix

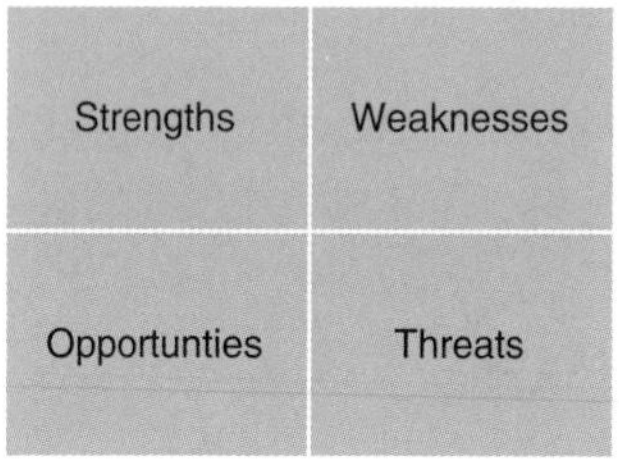

Strengths	Weaknesses
Opportunties	Threats

© Cengage Learning 2013

Exercises

Prepare a SWOT analysis for each of the following cases:

1. In *Case 1: Selling a Medicaid Managed Care Company*, evaluate Sunlight Health Plan to guide the company's decision to sell to another health plan or remain independent.

2. In *Case 2: Independent Medical Practices–Becoming Extinct?*, evaluate Woodland Family Practice within the context of selecting the best strategic option.

3. In *Case 3: Strategic Options Assessment for a Catholic Health System's Health Plan*, evaluate Healthy Lives and its relative market position.

4. In *Case 10: Managing Retail-Based Health Clinics: Financial Performance and Mission*, evaluate Pleasant Valley Medical Center's retail-based health clinic to help determine if Jeanne can turn the clinic around by the end of the fiscal year.

5. In *Case 19: Numbers and Degrees—Challenges for the Nursing Workforce*, read the Institute of Medicine's 2010 report, *The Future of Nursing: Leading Change, Advancing Health*, and evaluate MidMichigan Health within the context of its current RN workforce. The analysis should guide the organization's formulation of strategy to advance the current RN workforce for the health system.

Exercise 4

Mission Statements for Nonprofit and For-Profit Healthcare Organizations

Write a mission statement for the following healthcare organizations.

Concord Health System

Concord Health System (Concord) provides a comprehensive scope of services within the communities it serves. Founded more than 120 years ago, Concord has a long-standing tradition of providing patients with a single home for any medical care or need. Concord's system includes 20 acute care hospitals with 4,500 beds, 180 physician clinics, 15 assisted living and long-term care facilities, 10 hospice and home health programs, senior services, and many other health and educational services. The health system extends across four states in the Southeast with leading market reputations. Concord employs more than 45,000 professionals and it generated total operating revenue in the last fiscal year of more than $9 billion.

West Mountain Health

West Mountain Health (WMH) is a regional health insurance company that offers a broad range of health insurance and employee benefits products in two states in the Midwest. Established in 1970, the health plan is dedicated to helping its members improve their health and well-being. WMH offers health maintenance organization (HMO), preferred provider organization (PPO), and point-of-service (POS) insurance plans. The company also serves Medicare and Medicaid beneficiaries in its markets. WMH has membership of 1 million commercial, 75,000 Medicare, and 50,000 Medicaid members. The health plan has a healthcare network of more than 40,000 healthcare professionals, including primary care doctors and specialists, and more than 50 hospitals. Given its regional focus, the company faces intense competition from large national health plans. WMH employs more than 2,500 health professionals and its total revenue in the last fiscal year was nearly $2 billion.

Exercises

1. How might the mission statement be different if the organization is nonprofit or for-profit?

2. How would the governance be different between the nonprofit and for-profit organizations?

3. How would the strategic planning be different between the nonprofit and for-profit organizations?

Exercise 5 — Prisoners' Dilemma

The Prisoners' Dilemma (PD) is a classic game theory scenario in social science that provides an understanding of what governs the balance between competition and cooperation in social, business, and political situations. The PD involves a scenario where two people could cooperate and gain a positive result, but often don't because of how the payoffs are structured. The concept of the PD was developed by RAND Corporation scientists Merrill Flood and Melvin Dresher and was formalized by Albert W. Tucker.[1]

The traditional scenario involves two suspects who have been arrested by the police for a crime. The police have separated both prisoners and are interrogating them in separate rooms. The police visit each of them and offer them the same deal:

- If they both confess, each will receive a 5-year sentence.
- If one informs on the other and the other remains silent, then the informer will go free and the silent prisoner will receive the full 10-year sentence.
- If both stay silent, then the police can sentence both suspects to only 1 year in jail (i.e., not enough evidence without a confession for a longer sentence).

The scenario can be represented in a matrix.

		Prisoner B	
		Inform	Silent
Prisoner A	Inform	5 yrs for A, 5 yrs for B	0 yrs, 10 yrs
	Silent	10 yrs, 0 yrs	1 yr, 1 yr

© Cengage Learning 2013

Each prisoner must make the choice of whether to inform on the other suspect or remain silent, not knowing what choice the other prisoner will make. No matter what the other suspect does, each can improve his situation by informing on the other, thinking that the other will remain silent. Therefore, the dominant strategy for each, according to game theory, is to inform, which results in a worse outcome for both than if they both kept silent.

The PD has applications to business and economic strategy. It characterizes many economic decisions where there are only a few participants who have to decide individually, and where the outcome is influenced not only by their own decisions but by those of other participants. In business applications, the outcome or payoff in the PD scenario is the organization's profits. For example, take two health clinics selling a similar service and each clinic must decide on a pricing strategy relative to the other clinic, not knowing what choice the other clinic will make. The scenario can be represented in the following matrix.

	Health Clinic B	
	Low Price	High Price
Health Clinic A Low Price	$80 for A, $80 for B	$70, $120
High Price	$120, $70	$100, $100

The pricing strategy of the two health clinics can result in the following payoffs:

- If they both set a competitive low price (equivalent to each prisoner informing), each will make a profit of $80 per month.
- If one sets a competitive low price (i.e., think of it as undercutting the competitor) and the other has a higher price, then the clinic with the low price will win more customers from its competitor and increase its profit to $120 per month compared to only $70 for the other clinic.
- If both set a high price (equivalent to each prisoner remaining silent and cooperating), then they exploit their joint market power through the cooperation and each makes a profit of $100 per month.

Therefore, the dominant strategy for each health clinic is to undercut the other by setting a lower relative price (i.e., one prisoner informing on the other). The result of each clinic undercutting the other (or "cheating") is that both clinics end up making less profit than if they both cooperated.

Exercises

Using the PD framework described above, identify and explain the dominant business strategy in each of the following examples.

1. Consider two pharmaceutical companies (e.g., Pharma A and Pharma B) that have developed new drug therapies that have shown effectiveness in helping patients lose weight. The two drugs are considered equally effective with similar potential side effects. The companies must decide on their advertising strategy. An advertising strategy aimed directly to consumers is very expensive, with millions of dollars spent on television advertisements. Will the pharmaceutical companies advertise?

2. Consider two hospitals that have an excess number of underutilized beds. The hospitals are the only acute care providers in their market. The hospitals have a fixed cost expenditure associated with operating their inpatient beds. As their inpatient admissions increase, they can spread their fixed cost base over a larger number of utilized beds. If inpatient admissions remain low, they can reduce the number of beds operated by decreasing the level of staffing, resulting in a lower fixed cost base but also lower profit. The hospitals must consider their operating level and whether to restrict output, that is, reduce the number of beds operated. Will the hospitals reduce the number of beds operated?

3. Consider the same two hospitals in Exercise 2. The hospitals must decide on a pricing strategy for their inpatient admissions. A larger volume of inpatient admissions will lower the relative fixed costs per bed, resulting in higher profits. Will the hospitals cut prices?

4. Consider two surgery centers in a regional market that are considering purchasing the *da Vinci*® Surgical System (www.davincisurgery.com), which is a robotic platform designed to expand a surgeon's capabilities and offer a minimally invasive option for major surgery. The system claims to offer many benefits over traditional surgery including the potential for significantly less pain, a shorter hospital stay, faster return to normal daily activities, and better clinical outcomes. Each surgery center believes that if it can be the first clinic, and potentially the only clinic, in the market to have this system it will be able to increase patient volume and earn substantially higher profits, which ultimately will be necessary to justify its high cost. Will the surgery centers each buy a *da Vinci*® Surgical System?

5. In *Case 3: Strategic Options Assessment for a Catholic Health System's Health Plan*, Healthy Lives health plan faces a prisoners' dilemma in its regional market. The market is unique in that the HMO penetration is high, yet there are two major hospital systems, which both offer provider-sponsored health plans. St. Mary's Health System owns and operates Healthy Lives HMO, and University Medical System owns and operates Medical Care HMO. These two hospital systems have limited other HMO competition in the marketplace. As a result, the managed care rates that their respective hospitals (St. Mary's Hospital and University Hospital) have contracted with their own health plans have been set artificially low in order to maintain their relative market share among employer clients. Recall that the employers in this market have become more price sensitive, pressuring insurance premiums to remain low. As a result, the hospitals are earning a negative operating profit margin on a full-cost basis on business from their own health plans. As presented in Case 3, St. Mary's Health System is considering selling Healthy Lives. Describe the prisoners' dilemma for the two health systems in the regional market with respect to continuing to operate their respective HMO health plans. The scenario is represented in the following matrix to facilitate the discussion. What should the health systems do? What insights does the PD scenario provide with respect to the health systems' strategies?

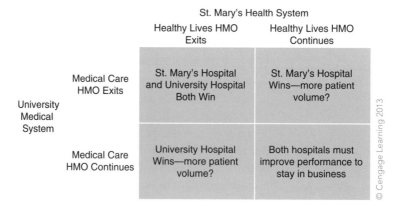

Reference

[1] Dixit, A., & Nalebuff, B. (2008). Prisoners' dilemma. In *The Concise Encyclopedia of Economics* (2nd ed.). Retrieved from http://www.econlib.org/library/Enc/PrisonersDilemma.html

Exercise 6

Business Wargaming

A business wargame is a role-playing exercise that is an adaptation of military wargaming to the business environment. Business wargaming helps a company with strategic, operational and tactical planning, and execution. It can apply to any nonprofit or for-profit organization that must execute on a business strategy to be successful. It helps a company anticipate the potential reactions of competitors and customers, as well as other uncontrollable events. The ultimate goal of the exercise is to help the organization significantly improve the probability of success for its strategy.

Business wargaming can be conducted at different levels of complexity. There are strategic management consulting firms, such as KappaWest Management Consultants, for example, that specialize in conducting business wargaming for organizations. The methodology summarized below offers a simplified version that can be easily conducted in an educational setting. For a formalized wargame format, refer to KappaWest Management Consultants White Paper, *Business Wargaming*.[1] In deciding whether to use a wargame approach to help an organization, the following criteria suggested by KappaWest can be used:

- The company's markets are saturating;
- New forces or competitors are entering the company's markets;
- The company's industry is undergoing significant change;
- The company's industry is consolidating;
- The company is evaluating alternative strategies and needs help in reaching a consensus as to which is best; and
- The company's market position is weakening.[1]

The key insights from a business wargame are gained through a mutual assessment of individual participants' experiences. During the wargame participants should reflect on what worked well in their strategies and what did not. They should seek to identify detailed insights into how and why they should adjust the initial business strategy, planning, and/or execution.

Wargame Teams

Establish at least four teams: company team, competitor teams, market team, and control team. In the classroom setting, each team should ideally consist of at least two students, with the exception of the competitor teams, in which an individual student may represent one competitor, and the control team, which will be comprised of the instructor and teaching assistants.

Company Team

The Company Team represents the organization in question that is executing on a strategic, operational, or tactical plan. The core of the business wargame revolves around this plan in question. The Company Team starts the game by making a decision and taking action on its plan.

Competitor Team(s)

There can be multiple teams representing different competitors to the company. Each Competitor Team should have a different mission and strategy; otherwise, the competitors can be represented by one team.

Market Team

The Market Team represents the amalgamation of market participants, primarily customers. The role of this team is to judge the relative attractiveness of the company's actions compared to its competitors and the market overall. The Market Team uses research and experience to respond to the actions of the company and competitors.

Control Team

The Control Team manages the wargame simulation and comprises the instructor and teaching assistants. The Control Team establishes the schedule, rules, and feedback among participants. This team should also adopt the role of any other stakeholders who might not be explicitly represented by other participants in the simulation, such as regulators, politicians, consumer advocacy groups, and other interest groups.

Business Wargame Simulation

The business wargame is a turn-based interaction, which is designed to simulate a certain timeframe in real life, such as a few months to several years. The first move of the game occurs in the present, based on all the data available at that time. Each move within the game represents a decision cycle. Each team meets in a separate location to discuss their primary objective and the strategy they will use to accomplish it. After reviewing their strategy, the Company and Competitor Teams make their decision and take the first action on their plan. For instance, these actions could include launching a new program, product, or service; entering a new market; establishing a business partnership; investing in new capacity; or conducting a new program or advertising campaign. The actions are documented and handed to the Market and Control Teams. All teams meet in a central location and then the Company and Competitor Teams present their actions to the industry (i.e., all teams in the game). The purpose of this presentation is to provide all parties with the same level of information on which they will base their next decisions. Following the presentation, the Market Team meets to provide feedback and judge the attractiveness of the actions of the Company and Competitor Teams. The Market Team will award relative scores for the Company and Competitor Teams. The Control Team will take these scores and translate them into metrics that can be used by the teams in the next round of decisions. For instance, the Control Team can calculate market shares, market sizes, sales volumes, customer volumes, profit margins, or other key performance indicators that might be pertinent to the scenario. This feedback from the Control Team will represent the starting point for each team to begin their next move.

A typical business wargame is organized around three moves, involving the equivalent of three days. On each day, the Company and Competitor teams meet in the morning, analyze the relative information from the Control Team, and prepare their actions, which include preparing for their presentations to the industry midday. In the afternoon, the Market Team reacts to the actions of the Company and Competitor Teams. In the evening, the Control Team calculates the impact of the relative scores and decisions made by the Market Team. The Control Team prepares a report for Company and Competitor Teams, which provides their relative key metrics. These reports serve as the starting point for the next move in the morning of the following day. During the sessions, the Control Team should monitor all communication among the teams. Communication is allowed among teams, much like in the real world, except in the wargame the communication should be channeled through email so it can be monitored by the Control Team. In addition, the Control Team can regulate what business actions and partnerships are permitted between the teams, similar to the role of regulators in the industry.

An alternative wargame schedule could involve the Company and Competitor teams meeting ahead of a class session and then giving their presentation to the industry at the next scheduled class session. After the class session, the Market and Control teams could meet and prepare their reports, which could be emailed to the Company and Competitor teams prior to the next scheduled class session (the following week, for instance). The Company and Competitor teams could then meet and prepare ahead of the next scheduled class session, and so forth.

Business Wargame Simulation Exercises

1. The industry in which your healthcare company operates is consolidating. Following the recently announced acquisitions by several of your competitors, there do not seem to be many good partners left. What should your company do?

   Examples of industries to consider for this scenario are the pharmacy benefit management (PBM) and the pharmaceutical industries. Small, regional players in these industries often lack critical mass and resources to effectively compete without a differentiated business strategy in an increasingly consolidated industry. A business wargame simulation of this scenario, for instance, could consist of the Company Team representing a small, regional PBM company and the Competitor teams representing several of the top three PBM companies (e.g., CVS Caremark, Express Scripts/Medco, Catamaran Corp. [SXC Health Solutions/Catalyst Health Solutions]). The Market Team would represent customers, including health plans and self-insured employers who contract with these PBMs for management of the pharmacy benefits for their members and employees. The Market Team would also represent the pharmaceutical companies and retail pharmacy chains that contract with the PBMs to supply the drugs at discounted prices. The Control Team would represent, among others, regulators from the Federal Trade Commission and state insurance commissioners. The Company Team would consider a business strategy in the face of a consolidating industry and how that strategy would be affected by its customers, distribution network of pharmacies, competitors, regulators, and other stakeholders.

2. Your company is planning the launch of a major new healthcare product or service. How will your launch strategy perform in the face of a much stronger competitor and the rapid development of a new alternative product or service design?

   An example to consider for this scenario includes the launch of a new drug therapy by a pharmaceutical company in the face of generic competition and new drug candidates under development by biotech companies. Another example includes the launch of a new narrow network HMO health insurance product by a health plan.

3. The business model in the industry in which your healthcare organization operates is changing. How will this change affect your organization? What should your organization do—embrace new models, defend the status quo, or some combination of both?

   An example to consider for this scenario is the accountable care organization (ACO) model. Under the Patient Protection and Affordable Care Act, the ACO model provides financial incentives for doctors and hospitals to deliver high-quality healthcare services to Medicare beneficiaries while keeping down costs. Although the legislation as written applies directly to the Medicare program, other healthcare organizations (hospitals, health plans, physician practices, and medical clinics) have been rapidly embracing similar accountable healthcare models in their markets for their member populations.

Reference

[1] Kurtz, C. J. (2007). Business wargaming. A Kappa White Paper. Retrieved from http://www.kappawest.com/WP_Business%20Wargaming.pdf

Exercise 7

Diplomacy and Engagement—Building the Afghanistan National Police Public Health System

CASE CONTRIBUTOR Douglas E. Anderson

A strong "Afghan Owned and Operated" civilian and military public health system along with military operations can result in helping the Afghan population become free of Taliban rule and selfish insurgent motives. The purpose of this real-world case study is to illustrate the need for a capabilities-based assessment approach to building a sustainable public health system. For example, it is easy to conduct a mass immunization program or identify training as a main solution. While these are good approaches, a capability-based approach assures long-term sustainment of health system development.

Situation

The past decade demonstrated that proper execution of public health diplomacy and engagement can be critical instruments to promote security, stability, and individual productivity. The opposite is true too. The U.S. military health sector development mission in Afghanistan (or Afghan) is helping the country's military and civilian health agencies overcome insurgent influence, strengthen local governance, and improve health by building a long-term health system capability. It's not easy. Several lessons have been relearned.

As part of the U.S. Military Counterinsurgency (COIN) strategy, military medical mentor (M3) teams were assigned to the Afghanistan National Security Forces (ANSF) to either build or improve the current health system in 2007. The ANSF consists of the Afghan National Army (ANA) and Afghan National Police (ANP). The ANA falls under the Ministry of Defense's (MoD) health system, while the ANP falls under the Ministry of the Interior's (MoI) health system. There was an informal agreement between the MoD and the MoI regarding the treatment of each other's personnel. Although ANP and their families are authorized care in MoPH hospitals, they are often turned away for security reasons. In fact, many die as a result. Despite their lack of resources and in some cases lack of utilization, all three organizations distrusted and preferred to compete with each other.

In 2008, Col. Anderson was assigned as the team leader for a 16-person military medical mentoring (M3) team for the ANP Surgeon General. He was the second team to continue with development. The team's responsibility was to assist the ANP on how to build their healthcare system for 82,000 police and 540,000 family members. Mentors were assigned to functional areas of the newly formed headquarters (HQ) team and hospital teams. More specifically, the objective was to build an Afghan Owned and Operated health system.

After an initial assessment, it was determined the ANP needed a public health capability covering the spectrum for the prevention and protection of personnel from disease, illness, and injuries while in garrison from the moment they arrive in an area of operations to the post-deployment setting. This capability required a surveillance, personal protective measures, and countermeasures program to reduce infectious disease threats, protect against environmental and occupational injury and illness, and prevention of non-battle injuries. The capability needed to incorporate infectious disease identification, monitoring, and reporting policies. Site and health risk assessment are key functions within the capability area to ensure the protection of forces in the garrison and deployed settings.

Although fragmented in terms of long-term planning and integration, basic Afghan Owned and Operated preventive health capabilities were slowly being developed. However, U.S. and NATO partners focused on near-term "feel good" initiatives. For example, routine vaccination of ANP and food safety inspections were done by the U.S. mentors. The roll-out of a number of educational posters and handbooks did not include the Afghans nor consider the cultural implications. While laudable, these efforts did not contribute to long-term sustainment or acceptance by the Afghans. For example, minimal effort was taken to build an overall action plan to track and certify progress. Training, much less a train-the-trainer program, was nonexistent. The medical supply distribution and equipment system was weak and riddled with corruption and hoarding. Finally, policies or reporting systems were never developed and ANP leadership was not involved in public health issues or aware of the impact on ANP readiness. Furthermore, U.S. solutions were being thrust upon the Afghans without their involvement, thus creating tension and resistance to change in an already tough situation.

This situation was further complicated by the lack of integration among the Ministry of Public Health (MoPH), MoD, and MoI leadership and the overall health system. Even more exasperating, the immediate U.S. military medical leadership had invested more time and resources in the MoD or ANA at the expense of the MoI's ANP. At present, the MoPH is not a key partner with the military mentoring teams because the MoPH oversees healthcare delivery for the Afghan civilian population, not the Afghan security forces. The MoPH should serve as a key counterpart ministry for the assigned military mentoring teams for the ANA and ANP. The MoPH should work closely with Afghanistan provincial authorities to ensure integration of U.S. military reconstruction, development, and training activities. It has been weak and sparse at best.

Even worse, the immediate U.S. military medical leadership did not see or care about the effects of a lack of ANP capabilities and integration of the overall health system, especially the public health sector, or take action to coordinate and negotiate the integration of public health capabilities for the ANP. As such, in many cases, Col. Anderson had to work outside the medical chain of command and rely on the overall U.S. ANP mentors to help the ANP. He also had to work extra hard at acquiring resources from the U.S. medical community. An Inspector General assessment later confirmed the lack of support in the U.S. military medical functional area.

Background

Although Afghanistan remained calm and stable in the 1960s–1970s, the health status of the people, especially women and children, was significantly lower when compared to other countries in the region. In 2002, the MoPH embarked on a new policy to create a Basic Package of Health Services (BPHS) template. This included preventive health services. The MoPH made the choice to restrict its role to (1) monitoring and evaluation; (2) coordination of donors' inputs; (3) strategic planning; (4) setting technical standards; (5) regulating the for-profit private sector; and (6) coordination and regulation of the Non-Governmental Organization (NGO) sector. Integration of the ANA and ANP health systems was not considered. A centralized coordination authority at the highest government levels or U.S. Ambassador levels did not exist. As of February 2008, Afghanistan still suffered from very high Infant Mortality Rates (IMR) (129:1000 live births), Under 5 Mortality Rate (U5MR) (191:1000 live births), and Maternal Mortality Rates (MMR) (16:1000 live births). One out of every five Afghan children dies before the age of 5. Life expectancy at birth is 47 years for men and 45 years for women.

The ultimate goal of the medical mentors is to enhance security by building an Afghan planned, owned, and operated health system. The mentors are there to help and advise the Afghans on how to create a sustainable capacity with Afghan solutions, not to import a U.S. or European system. Mentors are critically important. They are diplomats, advisors, and trainers often times offsetting the desires for Afghans to join the Taliban or other insurgents. Rebuilding the healthcare infrastructure of the ANSF is an important component of a COIN strategy to ensure gaining the trust of moderate Muslims in Afghanistan, denying terrorists a potential connection with a desperate populace, and giving hope and healing a chance. Military operations and defensive security actions continue to be sporadically coordinated with healthcare reconstruction activities so the resulting successes of combat actions are reinforced; however, coordination with health agencies and the military medical mentors is severely lacking.

Despite enormous strides since 2008, the ANSF still face a number of significant challenges, predominately in the areas of leader development, public health system stability, human resources management to include recruitment, training and discipline, hashish (20–40%) and opium use (10–15%) per ANP, and emergency management or response. The ANA are more developed than the ANP. The ANP have not received quality training, proper investment, or mentoring. As a result, the ANP do not have a fully functioning healthcare system or "official" inpatient capability. The medical requirements for 82,000 ANP and their 530,000 beneficiaries are significant. The current ANP healthcare system is Kabul-centric with only nine provincial health centers, an Academy clinic, and the Kabul National Primary Care Clinic. Future plans for the ANP include expanding the number of border, highway, and counter-narcotics police. A plan to build new clinics and recruit more health workers is in place.

The MoPH oversees all matters concerning the health of Afghanistan's population. It has a three-part mission: train, educate, and cure. Prior to 2005, almost six million Afghans had very little or no access to medical care. In addition, 50 of the country's 330 districts had no health facilities whatsoever. The 2009 public health goals are:

- Provide access to health care to all Afghans (85% of Afghans have access as defined by the U.N. criteria of walking 2 hours from their home to receive care);
- Improve maternal fetal health by decreasing female postpartum mortality and infant mortality;
- Increase vaccination rates throughout the country;
- Provide clean water to all citizens;

- Decrease childhood malnutrition rates; and
- Decrease the rates of infectious disease especially malaria, tuberculosis, and leishmaniasis.

The biggest challenge facing the MoPH is the lack of a proper mix of resources and poor integration. In some cases health facilities have been developed by international health donors, however, they are understaffed or not staffed at all. There is a shortage of both financial and human medical capital from which the MoPH can draw. The lack of a national tax base from which the government can obtain funds is a large obstacle in providing the Afghan citizens free health care as granted in the Afghan Constitution. The lack of money creates shortages of supplies and qualified medical staff but no shortage of graft. These shortages are felt hardest in the rural provinces. As the Afghan economy matures and is able to withstand taxation and as the current population of medical students graduates, the hope is that these problems will diminish.

Because the MoPH has no national source of revenue, it is reliant on international donations. This complicates coordination. As discussed above, the major donors are the World Bank, Arabian Development Bank, United States Agency for International Development, European Commission, and the KfW German Development Bank. In all instances, except with the European Commission, the money is managed by the MoPH, and health care is executed by NGOs. Therefore, the relationship between the NGOs and MoPH is robust but lacks integration and coordination.

Physician problems within Afghanistan also exist. First, there are not enough physicians in Afghanistan to manage the many clinics that have been established. This problem is more acute in the rural and war-torn areas. Second, there is a shortage of well-qualified physicians due to an educational system that unraveled during the Russian, warlord, and Taliban rules. Third, the pay physicians receive is quite low and other opportunities to earn a higher income exist, such as being an interpreter.

The ANP continue to take four to six times more casualties than ANA counterparts. Each ANP and family member deserves access to health care. Equally important, ANP commanders should expect fit and healthy ANP to include protection against disease and environmental threats, the ability to return patients to duty quickly, and efficiently take care of emergencies. A strong ANP preventive and primary care system integrated with the national health system allows ANP members to have confidence that their families are being taken care of, attracts high-quality applicants, and provides a solid foundation for retention.

Next Steps

The initial step to health system development especially when starting from scratch includes the employment of a capabilities assessment process. The team members must develop questions involving current policies and processes, organization, training, supplies and equipment, leadership skills, personnel, and facilities to guide the effort. After interviews, a capabilities assessment should result in a report assessing the (1) As-Is State, (2) To-Be State, and (3) Gaps. This results in a documented set of required capabilities (To-Be State).

For example, the capabilities assessment resulted in the need to assist the ANP in their long-term public health strategy. First, they need to be integrated with the ANA and MoPH. But how? New recruits require immunizations. Is this a priority? If so, why? There is no disease screening of ANP personnel and field sanitation is weak. Why is this important to operations? How are ANP commanders involved? Sanitation and hygiene programs are being improved; drinking water quality, food safety, and basic sanitation have also been stressed to improve the health of ANP troops and ensure minimal impact from diarrheal diseases. However, reports of food poisoning and anthrax cases are common. Why is this important? What Afghan solutions are required? An epidemiological surveillance system must either be developed or integrated.

Through epidemiological surveillance, ANP public health personnel will be able to monitor and sustain police strength and be capable of providing commanders with mission-critical health information as well as directing public health initiatives in the field. But will they? Is this a U.S.-driven solution? What training is required? The infection control system in hospitals, clinics, and units needs to be strengthened. Improved systems must be placed in highly populated ANP areas in order to minimize the spread of communicable diseases and deadly viruses (such as HIV and hepatitis). Are there written policies? With regard to hospital preventive health services, the lack of personnel across the ANP led to a dearth of trained preventive health professionals. Initiatives must be geared around developing training for the basics and comprehensive disease management. What's the long-term training solution?

Once the desired capabilities are developed, objectives and milestones must be implemented and monitored. While this may seem intuitive, it is actually difficult. First, since the job was to build sustainability and ownership, all actions had to be translated and accepted. Second, U.S. solutions are not necessarily the best solutions given the indigenous situation and culture. And finally, U.S. Mentors are deployed for six months; therefore, long-term solutions must be well managed and broken down into specific steps and continuity folders are required to keep the momentum going, otherwise stagnation and marginalization will set in.

Classroom Exercise

Divide the class into four groups, each addressing the questions below. Afterwards have a discussion about the different roles and outcomes for each group.

Group 1

1. What steps would you take to rebuilding a country's public health system? What would be your strategy? What type of leadership style would you employ to assure integration?

2. What public health system capabilities would you put in place first, second, third, . . . ?

Group 2

3. How would you make your advising and mentoring efforts more sustainable after you leave?

4. What guidelines or standards would you use for planning, assessing, and reporting?

Group 3

5. How would you coordinate your activities between the MoPH and ANSF (ANA and ANP)?

6. What would be your measures (input, process, and outcome) of success? How would you measure them? How would you hold the Afghans accountable?

Group 4

7. What is the mentor's role in public health diplomacy, engagement, and development? What skills are necessary to be successful?

8. How does leadership involvement facilitate or inhibit health system development? If you were Col. Anderson, what would you have done differently?